NEEDLE
IN THE
HEART

The House of Mad Eccentrics

NURSING and CARE at its FINEST

HARVEY GREENHALGH

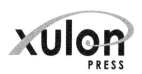

Needle In The Heart
The House of Mad Eccentrics
by Harvey Greenhalgh

Printed in the United States of America

ISBN 9781498419130

www.xulonpress.com

Raegan,

Thank you for
Caring.

Thank you for the effort
you made to win
this Book

Blessings,
—Be Great at all Things.

Jeremy

April 2015.

Dedication

This book is dedicated to my parents. To my Mother, Edith who successfully struggled with five children, beginning when our Father, Eric was still away in the Royal Air Force in World War Two. They brought all the children up to be a success in each of their lives. Times were difficult but slowly the family moved to larger homes as the children grew and matured.

I had been a sick child during the formative school years and had missed so much early education; my Dad Eric spent countless hours on countless hours with me, teaching me the basics of Math, Science, History, Geography and English, even teaching some of his most favourite Poetry.

Whatever and all the scholastic achievements I received, I dedicated them to my Dad. For it was he who spent those vast numbers of hours, encouraging me to keep going when I wanted to stop. It was not easy for him, but he did it for me.

So to Edith my Mum, who cared for my many times of sickness, and to my Dad who cared about my education, and therefore my future life.

Thank You both for your Love, Patience and being role models.

Acknowledgements

All the majestic elements of this story are factual. The Places, Towns, Regional Medical Centers and the names of all these amazing characters I have changed for privacy needs.

Although more than half a century has skipped on by all these grand events are indelibly imprinted onto my memory. I can still smile or even shed a tear in recapturing those truly wonderful moments for this book.

Thank You Matron, Hospital Sisters, Staff Nurses, those Eccentric, Bizarre and Other Physicians all, my Student Nursing colleagues and all my Patients from that wondrous hospital complex, the Fortress!

I want to thank my dearest wife Jane for the time she labored over my written words and then processing them into pages, then making the changes and corrections, it seemed dauntless but through her patience she prevailed.

My son David read my first few chapters', and then later did an in-depth review of my work, which were still in need of finer corrections to make the 'flow' and 'prose' and to keep the story moving, but more specifically to keep the story a personal one from my unique perspective. His advice and critique was seasoned and I am grateful to him.

Table of Contents

Introduction

I was a sick child. I probably had every bug, disease and surgery that a classroom of kids all had put together. So in England, I failed the *eleven plus* exam, which would have taken me into higher education. Instead I went to a school teaching technical skills. However, by age fifteen, the compulsory age for leaving, I had begun to achieve academically rising to the top of the three classes in that final year. The credit was not my own, but goes to my father who was my ever-patient coach and encourager.

By then it was too late for a finer more classical education. I was very good at technical engineering drawing so off I went to become a draftsman at a large engineering company that, amongst other things built jet aircraft.

Sadly for me this apprenticeship required completing five years learning how to be an engineer. Tragically for this huge engineering company in my second year I had two 'accidents'. The first was with a massive Cincinnati milling machine and the second was with a complex lathe machine. These were two wonderful machines in the right hands, but for me, I successfully destroyed them. The apprentice foreman took evasive action from future machine devastation and 'promoted' me to the jig and tool room stores, away from dangerous machines.

It very clear to me, after six months in the tool-room stores, that they had no plans to put me back on any machines. So I carefully interpreted their actions, and resigned. My dreams of being a fine draughtsman with a decent wage disappeared from my view.

But I knew where I was going! Two things came together at the same time to give me a totally different vision for my life. I had been in the Boy Scouts for six years and was on the St. Johns ambulance brigade first aid competition team. My team and I were very good; we won almost all our competitions against local, town, then regional teams doing these 'mass accident' scenarios where we would apply our first aid knowledge and skills. I knew fractures, bruises and bleeders and how to treat them.

During my last year of school I had two surgeries on my left arm. I sustained the injury whilst playing football. The injury came from some over aggressive center forward as he swung his right boot to kick the ball, he missed, hitting my left arm and wrist, which immediately went to protect my manhood, so by a split second my left arm became their protector and paid a painful price.

This stocky lad's boot smashed into my left forearm. Nothing broke, but it was extremely painful. Months later the pain in that left forearm was diagnosed to be osteomyelitis, or a Brodie's Abscess and it required immediate surgery. This meant instant hospitalization, and into the orthopedic Ward I entered as a patient. Once the surgery of opening up the bone, draining the infection, and pumping in some Sulphonamide drugs was complete, I started taking careful note of the hospital Ward's routine, realities and possible romances. The operation had to be repeated four months later since the pain had become too intense and unbearable, so back once more into the Orthopaedic Ward for another surgery I went. With the operation completed and healing progressing again I was now becoming a keen observer and mentally recording this hospital world around me and I was really enjoying it. I knew could do this.

At fifteen I left school. Surgeries had recently been done and my apprenticeship looked liked I was on track to become a draughtsman. At sixteen, by the end of that year I had mangled those two expensive engineering machines, and made the decision that I was failing in this apprenticeship so I needed to change the direction of my life. Within a week of resigning as an apprentice-engineering draughtsman I applied to our local hospital to become a Cadet Nurse and was accepted. In England, this programme had been established to give men and women who had not yet reached the official age of eighteen, the age to begin as a student nurse, to become cadet nurses. I liked this clever idea! Those who could not take the lengthy hours, and all the menial housekeeping jobs required of a cadet nurse, would drop out before becoming student nurse, neat and cost effective.

Those who 'made the grade' and possibly enjoyed it, went from Cadet Nurse to Student Nurse. That was my pathway into nursing and medicine and I would do it all over again. Indeed, the Fortress was waiting for me.

Preface

The Fortress

The Hospital, its Inhabitants and all who Dwell there

Growing up under the long dark shadows of this black stone structure that dominated the towns' skyline, I believed, still held the power of an ancient Fortress. Built in 1708 on the highest hill surrounding our town its bleak overwhelming, ominous presence proved its appearance and character by having more turrets, spires, ramparts and protective outer walls than all the other churches, ancestral homes, town clock tower and the Town Hall put together!

My home was down the hill from this towering Fortress where its presence dominated everyday life itself. The trees, and a lake in the park just a short distance away were the only barrier between the Fortress and my home. Even from some distance away and even clothed in its dark shadows its eerie back cold nature of its stone told a story of days of very long ago, even the multitude of its windows appeared dark, drab and unseeing.

An uncle of mine had worked at one of the towns' cotton weaving mills and in my later life I had teased him by saying he was responsible for turning the Fortress and other older buildings into masses of black brick and stone from the constant dirty smoke that belched from the chimneys of his cotton mill.

Over the years the black sooty smoke billowing from the towns cotton mills chimney stacks', of which there were many, had left their indelible mark on many aging buildings, so that by the 1950's this architectural wonder was an ebony black color of smooth granite stone. Perhaps even more forebodingly eerie during the winter's dark cloudy and moonless nights, was when the huge trees surrounding its grounds creaked and rustled in the blustery winds.

This architectural Fortress wonder was my hospital, I was going to study there, so now it belonged to me, and it was losing its darker foreboding characteristics. Over the years, especially through the early era of the Victorian period it has been home to the *poor house*, and alternatively called the *work house*, where the needy, destitute, orphans, beggars and the sick would come seeking food and shelter. Some, those strong enough, would work on the farms or the agricultural lands surrounding the Fortress. By end of the Victorian period and early years of the nineteenth century a huge laundry and an even bigger cookhouse, had been created in the bowers of our Fortress.

This hospital Fortress was surrounded on two sides by lovely grazing fields of green grass, where a dairy herd of cattle lazily ate their fill in one field. Whilst In another field, small horses and the huge carthorses ran with each other, and below that field another with grazing sheep. Always so picturesque and peaceful. The tall trees between the pasturelands were powerful old oaks and between them were the mature Chestnut trees. On sunny days when the gentle westerly breeze took the branches and waved them in harmony, it appeared from a distance that the leaves from all the trees created a moving landscape, almost moving the Fortress from side to side in a mystical and musical way.

The main access to our hospital was through one main gate where everyone had to pass its stony portals to reach any of the many buildings in existence in the 1950's, even then, uniformed guards would stop all the cars to ask their destination. The guard at the gated visitors entrance tipped his hat respectfully but also wanted to know the destination of each person, a pleasant chap with a lot of places to remember! Well, through this entrance for the first time is where my story begins. Later, I quickly learned of a short cut by the side of the fields, I could get access through an old decrepit small wooden gate, and it saved a ton of time!

Besides the massive main hospital building there where buildings with architecture from the Victorian era to the present day 1950's. They included a huge Geriatric facility. A home to over 200 long-term care male and female residents, with the myriad aging dilemmas, some of them had been there for over 8 year's never leaving the building. Amazing that these patients never had any bedsores, a great tribute to great Nursing Care.

Then there was the Psychiatric hospital that shared the joyless, ominous dark features of the main Fortress. This building was home to both sexes and accommodated acute psychiatric diagnoses as well as long term care patients, who almost seemed to be part of the building itself, some patients perhaps, hiding in the nooks and crannies of their shadows flitting mysteriously across hallways and down darkened corridors.

There were two relatively newer buildings in the furthest corner of this huge domain. Both built originally with a lovely red brick but now gently clothed with a grey coating of chimney grime rather than the black chimney soot of our turreted Fortress.

The larger of the two red brick buildings was a two-story Student Nurses Home. These residents were the female Student Nurses, generally for those who had come from other parts of Britain, Ireland particularly, as well as French, German and Austrian ladies. The male Student Nurses were forbidden to go anywhere near the Nurses Home! We never knew why, but supposed was it 'good manners' not to get close? However, the male nurses searched for ways to get close anyway!

Near the nurses home was our Pediatric hospital, and always the male Student Nurses loved their assignments to 'PEDS', since it gave them the possibility of getting closer to the Student Nurses Home with its hundreds of curtained windows, and visions of those lovely ladies even in their stark nurses uniforms.... or possibly without them.

Adjacent to the PEDS building was the Nursing Education Center but it actually looked more like an instantly fabricated farm shed than a place of higher education. Its two classrooms both of which overlooked the fields of the grazing cattle and sheep in one field and carthorses in the other field. Sadly, no windows looked directly towards the Nurses Home. Probably not planned that way, but it did mean all the male students' concentration was on their subject study. Even the tutor or a lecturing consultant physician, keeping our attention away from the Nurses Home by explaining exactly why we should always use our God given 'senses' of vision, touch, hearing and smell. The Tutor taught the idea of our taste sense as a light hearted jest and discarded as not very wise to pop your finger in your mouth (after supposedly dipping it into urine, then switching fingers) unless you were desperate for a *'comforting suck'*, as the pediatric consultant would also gleefully share. I remember groaning at this idea

This lovely old complex of aging stone and granite with its colourful history was a vital hub of activity of scurrying ambulances, hectic and jostling visitors. Cars always desperate to find a less than adequate parking spot, as well as a constant stream of staff-nurses and students in their heavy woolen navy blue capes, with their white wing folded caps, or caps with frills around the cap edges declaring seniority. These nursing caps in a variety of shapes from those worn by the Matron, or Sisters all the way down the scale to the first year Student Nurses. Their caps looked like ancient flying machines especially when carefully starched and folded, then pressed, ironed and finally pinned into their hair with great skill and balance.

Remarkably those caps stayed in place no matter what circumstances were encountered. Remarkable too since these *angels of mercy* had to walk from the Nurses Home to whichever part of the hospital they were working. Even through the inclement weather of what seemed like gale force winds or driving cold rain that battered this hill top monument, and the nurses caps stayed attached to their hair. Those girls braved the raging rain and blustery blizzards of all seasons whilst hanging on to their nursing caps that rather would have been high-flying kites.

Sometimes it may have looked to me like I was looking into the face of history, when before me, was the power and authority of 'the Fortress Nation'-the Matron, Sisters, the Staff Nurses and a league of Consulting Physicians and Doctors of every Specialty.

Awe inspiring or fiercely frightening to a first year Student Nurse who has just learned how the dramatic lines of authority were derived which meant that she or he was barely above the level of the waiters in the Doctor's Dining Room, but what a challenge and opportunity.

CHAPTER 1.

The Power Brokers

Those Starched Ladies in Navy Blue

The Matron's uniform was deep dark green colour. It was a fairly simple one-piece dress with a high collar that fit closely around her neck. Her Matronly cap could have duplicated for a birthday cake with a lovely starched lace ribbon crowning its peak. At the end of her long sleeves were beautifully & carefully cultured starched lace cuffs, her dress was belted simply and whether the Matron was large or small in stature never really mattered because her's was the highest of powers. A visit to the Matron for some discovered misdeed would send a sense of anxiety creeping across your life and future.

In truth, and in looking back at the Matron I had, she was as authoritarian as any might expect, but on meeting her face-to-face on one event for a reported immature offense that needed a disciplinary action (mimicking the chanting of the Priest in the main hospital corridor—after he had caught myself and my friend), changed that view.

Coming into her office, a large well lit and stylishly furnished room with two chairs directly in front of her huge desk, the complaining Priest was already sitting in one of the chairs. The Matron asked me to introduce myself then offered me the empty chair, and when I had sat down she asked the Priest to explain why I had been offensive to him. He told his story of my inappropriate attitude and chanting which he did not like. The Matron, listening to him but looking at me with a careful gaze, finally asked the Priest if he would leave and allow her to discipline me, the guilty party. After the Priest was gone, the Matron sighed a deep sigh, leveled her eyes back into mine and for a few seconds said nothing which had me fearful of some terrible penalty, but finally she smiled kindly and said simply, *"Don't do it again"*!

I left her office a new man, deciding never to get caught in the future, but my admiration for this Lady was forever changed.

However, I recognized quickly in the minute-by-minute position of authority were the Ward Sisters in their very recognizable Navy Blue Uniforms. Not a kindly religious sisterly order but the power and the punch of company sergeant majors, their measured words spoken in a variety of usually threatening almost thunderous demands were meant to have the listener like myself, obey instantly without wetting my pants or becoming a nervous wreck on the spot.

Remarkably, even the medical students, housemen, residents and mighty consultants, as well as everyone else wisely respected these navy blue uniformed 'battle axes' as their commanding officer. The Matron had given them total authority over lives, and my life changed under this voice of great authority and power, eventually under this leadership I would become an excellent Nurse.

The local population having their grand array of diseases, rare illnesses, mental and emotional dilemmas, pregnancies and a wild variety of major or minor traumas would come and visit us, hoping for recovery or a resolution of every ache and pain then return to life in this aging northern, cotton mill town.

The Students, Shining Knights and Maidens of the Court

The life and soul of every hospital was its Student Nurses. These were the days when the hospital was a teaching institution as well as the medical facility itself. The three-year programme throughout Britain from Student Nurse to State Registered Nurse was identical.

If one hospital lacked any particular department as perhaps, obstetrics or psychiatry then Student Nurses would simply rotate to a hospital in the region that had that specialty. This seemed to work beautifully giving the Student Nurses a change of senior nursing staff, physicians and of course some new lovely Student Nurses faces to admire.

However, before becoming a student nurse, some hospital districts had a specialized programme for 17 year olds who wanted to become nurses, but were still too young the programme was called 'Cadet Nursing'. I was one who took advantage of this opportunity for it was a clever idea which guaranteed that anyone who wanted to become a student nurse would be thrust into the hospital world of hygiene, actually working to keep the Wards as clean as possible doing the scrubbing, dusting, sweeping and all the extra house keeping duties normally done by the Ward Orderlies. These were some of the duties I performed as a Cadet Nurse and I got a small salary for it, but it was hard work and it seemed endless, it was certainly a great introduction to the world of nursing.

There was a strict adherence to seniority protocol. First year nurses, lowest on the totem pole would almost- but not quite, bow to the second year nurses, and they in turn paid homage to the wiser third year nurses who clearly knew how the system really worked, or at least how far they could go in any matter without engendering the barks of the power elite those ladies in Navy Blue!

Life was good and I began to learn so much especially since I actually enjoyed the hard grind, and a commitment of my soul for those three years. But there were times of frivolity, even times of fun, wonderful humor and side splitting laughter, sometimes these times were self created from the events before us. In other instant circumstances that were incredibly remarkable, perhaps unrepeatable were times watching our mad eccentric consultants with their rather odd antics.

The female Student Nurses outnumbered the male students, but not by many in all general hospitals. In the 'mental' hospitals, usually those hospitals dealing with diseases or anomalies of the brain rather than the acute psychotic breaks or grave anxiety disorders, male and female Student Nurses had equal numbers. Male nurses wore the white coats and unless you could read their nametags there was no determining first, second or third year student status, we probably all looked the same white-coated starchy lot.

In designating the levels of seniority for the female nurses, their uniforms were more colourful and had more flair. There was the light blue of the dress with short sleeves, which had a white puffy lace cuff just above the elbow; their bid-apron was the familiar white with its highly starched cotton. Occasionally some of the nurses pinned a watch with a second hand on to the upper left corner of their bib, this to make counting a radial pulse more easily.

It was their white 'flying wings' nursing cap that had their rank, with one, two or three dark blue strips to the left side on the broad band where the whole cap was folded back. There was actually a grand work of art involved in it's folding since it too was highly starched. Ironing could take up to 10 minutes to create this sculptured aerial masterpiece.

Perhaps as might be determined, all the first year nurses got the less exciting and more tedious, dirtier jobs to do. Even before the day shift got underway we had a brief report from 'miss thunder' (our nursing sister), who gave one or two Student Nurses from each group their appropriate report and sent us off to do the real tasks of thoroughly scrubbing the stainless steel bed pans, urinals, kidney dishes and measuring containers of various sizes. When they were done and mirror shining clean, into the larger of the two boiling, steaming sterilizers they would go. All the instruments and utensils would boil for an hour in the sterilizer to 'kill the bugs'; this was our sterilizing procedure. I remember doing this noisy job, due to the stainless steel banging together in the huge sinks, every morning.

Then every morning came the sharpening of all the stainless steel needles, now this was bringing home the skill of the ancient blacksmith and the royal armorer! I could see myself becoming a fine swordsman. Each needle went through a time honored process as each needle, whether hypodermic, intra dermal, intramuscular, intravenous or frighteningly, to the huge spinal needles. By the time I or anyone else had finished sharpening them they looked like a skilled swordsman could have used them to defend his honor. The needles were then attached to a clean glass syringe and the needle was thoroughly irrigated to make sure it was completely clear of any debris perhaps from a sliver of skin or fat tissue that may have lodged inside as the needle was removed from a patient. Once cleaned and clear the next vitally important job was to make quite sure the needle was very sharp-not the slightest suggestion of a 'barb', a blunt or needle point turned inwards, at its tip since it was the barb's on the end of needles that caused the extra pain due to the barb tearing tissue, rather than the clean, sharp and precise *stick* that was required. No 'use it once' then discard it that was a future luxury. Almost everything was cleaned and reused except the surgeon's scalpel, I firmly believed our sharpening could never match the manufacturers super-sharp edge, but if asked we would have tried!

The swordsman's sharpening duties fell to the male nurses especially the first year nurses and they, like I relished this task of sharpening and removing the barbs. What kind of sin, human or otherwise was it that created the barbs in the first place? It was also unclear how many needles were sharpened till there was nothing left to sharpen and eventually so very short they were cast out into a mysterious needle pit to be rejected and thus rust away.

I remember on one occasion, one of the Internal Medical Consultants coming into the Medical Ward one late afternoon to do a 'Spinal Tap' to draw some Cerebro- Spinal fluid from a patient. The Resident physician had tried many times and abandoned his efforts as too difficult and so called in the expert, the chief to do the procedure, and he arrived puffing and panting, wondering why his junior colleague could not succeed. Everything was ready and laid out for the procedure at the patients bedside, the Great Man had gowned and gloved, and he placed the sterile towels over the patient, now in position, and more towels on the bed. With his gloved hand he found the space between the vertebrae he wanted, he turned, picked up the glass syringe with its 3 inch spinal needle found the space again and plunged the needle into the bony spinal column and the patient howled a mighty noise-surprising everyone there!

The Consultant, withdrawing the needle felt the needles tip and lo and behold it had a barb at its end! He shouted a word of profanity and threw the syringe with its needle to the floor. Surprisingly the needle impaled itself into the wood floor and the syringe wobbled from side to side like a leaf in the wind. The Doctor said, "*Oooops*", as the needle and syringe landed one inch from his right foot. But the barb problem created an inquest on who may have been responsible, no one was ever held accountable, everyone sharpened the needles even sharper thereafter.

The second year nurses had the responsibility of the evening and night shifts on all the Wards. This was the place to be, and I was certainly as excited as everyone else, for it was on these shifts, no Sisters roamed their domain at nights. Almost everyone looked forward to their stint of independence, not quite freedom, but almost.

Night shift began with a report of how the patients had made it through the day, what to expect through the night, who may finally 'expire', and who may even present a spectacle of sorts. Like an erupting aortic aneurism!

The blackness of night within the Fortress Hospital on the different Wards, I found had its own sense of mystery for now I was in charge; as second year Student Nurses we knew what we were doing. We were given this independence, to assess and make our own critical judgments, to hopefully act with wisdom and probably with some bravado.

Of course the Night Shift Sister would do her rounds of all the Wards, ask if she could help and get a brief report on any difficult or problem patient, and if necessary we could call the Resident or Intern Houseman who was on duty sleeping in his 'call room' in the hospital for that night.

For myself and the other male nurses, we were really happy to have more freedom to move around the different floors of each hospital division, mainly to check out which of the female nurses we may be happy to see, or not to chat with. Chat light-heartedly with or, as presented an opportunity to sit with and explore both the nights event's or to propose a meeting sometime later. The possibilities seemed endless! Pub lunch or get together, local football match on a Saturday afternoon, or meet late evening at the towns' main boulevard, where all the local buses began and ended their routes; to buy one of those steaming, huge hot roasted potatoes and loaded with salt, that were for sale from the man with his horse and roasting oven on his cart, on cold weekend nights.

To me, nights seemed Florence Nightingale-like, lots of patients with surgical wounds, bandages, legs or arms-sometimes both held aloft on overhead pulleys, wounds being drained, blood transfusions in progress and medications all handed out! On the small desk in the middle of the Ward was a solitary low light. Remembering that a full Ward could have up to 12 to 14 beds down each side facing each other across the Ward, then in the middle a further 4 or 5 beds length ways from the far end of the Ward towards the entrance door.

The Ward Sister's office was located in the corridor at the Wards entrance but during our night hours her office was dark, quiet, at peace, and what a joy it was for me, for now I was in command of this breathing mass of sickly bodies the Ward was truly mine.

As my own experience increased I could listen to the breathing patterns of each patient and learned to recognize which poor souls were on their last legs, or based on their poor prognosis, torturous respirations and hear the fading moments of their straining lungs desperate for air.

Cardiac arrest 'crash carts' had not been yet invented, nor defibrillators, they were visions of things to come, but we did have our emergency tray. Even if the tray did not exist we could very quickly create one. The sterilizer, syringes, needles, kidney dishes, flat instrument trays and a variety of catheters, red rubber I.V. tubing, dressings, and bandages were within arms reach and the drug cabinet close by.

As bright shining Student Nurses we had learned that the drug Coramine was of wonderful cardiac stimulant, and since there was a small supply of Coramine in glass ampoules, in the medicine cabinet and there were 10ml. or 20 ml. glass syringes with the choice of needles, long spinal needles like swords or at least like a fine stiletto dagger. With these instruments I could provide instant cardiac action, perhaps even Heroic and life saving.

Sitting at my desk in the middle of the Ward, or doing my frequent patient rounds I always had an ear open for those with labored breathing, or occasionally seeing the pink bubbly froth that came from lungs drowning in their own pulmonary edema secretions, and I was ready should their breathing stop. An oxygen catheter hissing the hopeful life giving air, now producing no life sustaining benefit, and all the physical signs of life had ceased. Placing my well worn stethoscope on the chest brought only silence to my ears, no breath sounds, no heart beat heard, life was ebbing rapidly away, no viable thread of pulse at wrist or carotids on the neck. Now I bounded into action, sprinted to the medicine cabinet, I attached the spinal needle to the sterilized 20 ml syringe, then snapped open the neck of the glass vial then syphoned the Coramine into the syringe, grabbed some cotton wool swabs, poured Methylated Spirits on the swabs and ran to the immobile patient.

I remember doing this several times over my three years and always with great urgency and with my own Adrenaline pumping and rushing me on, then with one hand I swabbed and cleaned the left side of the chest and with the fingers of other hand found a spot between the ribs over the heart *and plunged this spinal needle-in-the-heart.*

To be certain I was in the heart I drew up on the syringes plunger so I could see that bright red blood, and with this certainty, pushed this cardiac stimulant drug into this probable stationary heart.

Once the whole amount was injected, and as I had been taught that a powerful shock to the heart muscle might achieve the electrical cardiac response to start a heart beat again, so with my clenched fist I pounded on this poor patient's sternum then vigorously rubbed over the area in a circular motion. I repeated this 5 or 6 times, waiting a few seconds between the pounding to listen with my stethoscope for any signs of a heat beat. Many Coramine injections into the heart were used in these valiant attempts, but we never had any life giving success in spite of trying so hard.

The later modern medicine drug, Lasix became a remarkable diuretic had not yet appeared, so the pulmonary edema drama left us all feeling powerless, but yes we did attempt this wondrous intra-thoracic 'needle in the heart' treatment!

There was never any need to do a post mortem on these patients since the physicians had diagnosed these patients and the obvious needle mark above the heart that we had left were never questioned by the pathologist. We were Student Nurses, and we were in command.

This needle-in-the-heart attempt at bringing someone back to life was the best effort at resuscitation that we had. When we were quite certain that our patient was in the last throes of life, whatever drugs we were using, and with the flow of oxygen from the huge green O2 cylinders through those red rubber-tubing catheters, or the oxygen mask; then perhaps that almost heroic needle deep into heart was the very last chance of living. This was 'Nursing' and I felt a deep sense of satisfaction.

Years and years later that *'needle into the heart'* routine may have been the unrecognized precursor for doing that incredibly dramatic procedure in the Casualty Department of cracking a chest. That by making an incision through the chest wall to actually crack open then spread the ribs apart, to physically hold the heart and 'pump' it. That is a life saving cataclysmic event of enormous proportions especially when it's successful, for the assistant or on-looker this awe-inspiring vision would never to be forgotten, the progression of modern medicine continues.

Clinic's, a Spot of Bleeding and Pandemonium

The Fortress Hospital had simple titles for its different Wards and clinics, no complicated names just the simple Pediatrics, Medical, Surgical, 'OB', 'GYN', Casualty, Operating Room, Clinics and the Mental Ward, no kinder references like Psychiatry. There was a fairly large Geriatric hospital on the grounds and a constantly busy Clinic area where on different days of the week, it would be taken over by the specialties of medicine, surgery, obstetrics and so on. This would bring together the medical staff of the consultant, his senior and junior housemen and a medical student or two. If a diagnosis was unclear or perplexing then a more specific investigation was needed. When that happened, the consultant would refer to the regional hospital center in a much larger city where the endocrinologist, epidemiologists, infectious disease specialists, or other key doctors practiced. The Casualty department adjoined the Clinics via a lengthy green tiled corridor. There was a large waiting room with old oak benches, hard as a rock to sit on, and since the examining rooms almost surrounded the waiting room, everyone in pain who wanted immediate attention cried or moaned in gay abandon. At times it was the sound of a symphony or an orchestral hall of a cacophony of loud protesting voices, and like pandemonium breaking loose, all wondering why they had to wait so long and why the benches were so hard and miserable to sit on!

One had to be bleeding, *really* bleeding or with a face of purple cyanotic colour and on your last breath of life to get priority treatment, the queue was the rule. This was a great place to work on your patience *skills.*

Occasionally I would borrow one of the nursing orderlies from the orthopedic Ward to come and demand quiet, his voice was more authoritative than mine. This was Joshua and he was proudly from Barbados, his skin a shiny black ebony, his rippling muscles showed prominently under his green orderly uniform smock and his 167 lbs. small frame of about five foot six was attention getting! He had served in the British Army for 21 years in the Royal Army Medical Corps, ending his career as a sergeant. When he demanded quiet from this seemingly unruly waiting room, he got it and quickly. Perhaps it was his lovely black face that was adorned by a shock of pure white hair! But whatever it was everyone including the children listened peace had come again.

Meet One Mad Eccentric, our Surgical Chief Consultant

If you met our chief surgical consultant somewhere other than the hospital or at his surgery, then you might have assumed he was a farmer. Actually, he probably would have been a great gentleman farmer.

His mop of hair never looked combed or cared for. He wore this once elegant brown tweed suit, now wearing thread bare at the elbows and collar and desperately in need of cleaning and repair. In harmony with this was his aging green tweed tie that was always in a perfect knot, but sported a variety of noticeable stains in a palette of colours. Brown probably from gravy, red from tomato ketchup, a whitish-yellow, possibly from a custard dessert and a collection of darkish yellow stains, certainly of a Coleman's mustard variety. It was always joy for me to see if I could spot a new stain adorning that tie or jacket. Adding to all of this was his mustache, also straggly and unkempt but it created a further joyful puzzle for everyone to try and decide what he had for breakfast that day. Crumbs of toasts or bread, tiny pieces of cereal, scrambled or boiled egg bits hung precariously in his hairy mustache. Everyone doubted that he ever looked in a mirror, owned a comb or hairbrush. I supposed that his wife had totally given up on trying to keep him in the style of dress that a chief surgical consultant should be attired! He wore Brown Boots, and they too were stained. An oddity in itself, Consultants should be wearing the finest English leather dress shoes-all the others did!

This man was indeed in the arena of *odd* or more gently described he was simply eccentric or bizarre or whatever category he might fit into but he was certainly a brilliant surgeon, and he was the Chief.

He bore his name, David Peter Alexander without any air or graces although he came from a line of wealthy landowners and besides which his father was a well recognized Cardiologist in his own right, so the Alexander dynasty had blood and guts in their family history and in its foreseeable future.

Doctor David Peter Alexander was the hospital's regional Chief Surgical Consultant, besides having his own private clinic surgery in the more affluent part of this old town, which was located on the ground floor in a huge well kept Victorian mansion surrounded by lovely Rhododendron bushes and a perfectly mowed lawn.

His car too was in complete harmony with his daily dress. It was a large saloon car and the only time it ever got cleaned was when it rained! We did not need to look further than his car to know if it had just rained. The window-wipers kept the front windows fairly clean at least the two arches created by the wipers moved away the mud, dust and in winter, the snow. Truly this machine of his was an ongoing work of art. After 6 months of grime accumulation anyone looking at the car could never guess its original colour.

He did buy a new car every year; it was probably cheaper than paying for car washes I thought, and why waste the time waiting for the car to be cleaned? On those new car occasions one of us might be brave enough to ask him what model he had chosen.

As a group of male nurses we kindly wanted to call him 'Lord Alexander', for we loved his entire array of quirky characteristics, but as the code of ethics clearly stated he was Mr. Alexander. For some strange reason the title of Mr. was only given to the chief consultants. The much more familiar title of 'doctor' was for the retinue of junior physicians. The Resident Housemen and the other consultants would always use the higher ranking, respectful title of 'Mr.'

Our 'Lord Alexander' seemingly being unaware of everyone or unconcerned of what anyone else might think including his wife, about his attire from that well worn brown tweed suit to his artistically stained brown boots and now creatively coloured green tweed tie. He would attend our more festive hospital events from graduations to the yearly, and very well attended Christmas Party and Ball in this same suit and boots, amazing!

I know we discussed at length, that if we were to return in three years from now, he would not have changed any item of clothing. The only possibility of change in him was that his hair and mustache may be trimmed, but again that was only a maybe.

Our lectures with him were always events to be remembered. Whether we had one, two or more hours of lectures they were always memorable. They were usually more memorable than they were educational, not from any lack on his part but from the bizarre and absent-minded nature of his lectures.

The lectures were held in the red brick education center with its windows overlooking the farmers' field. Whether or not our dear Lord Alexander loved animals or not we never knew, but we listened to his words of medical and surgical wisdom on a myriad of subjects. Such as, 'Why it was appropriate to flood the body with antibiotics'? Or 'Do an exploratory abdominal surgery using the greatest incision possible for unobstructed access'. He moved away from his central podium to the classroom windows and watched cows lazily chewing grass, or the horses with their folds in the fields, all of this whilst continuing his lecture and seemingly unaware of us, his students hanging on to his well refined Cambridge accent and his tales of surgical adventures.

Perhaps the most amazing and certainly quite funny, was his ability to lecture for almost an hour whilst finding nothing to see through the windows would then concentrate on a fly buzzing around a light fixture or crawling across the ceiling. He would not just follow the flying insect from one spot to the next with his eyes, but If necessary, and more often than not he would transverse the classroom moving between our desks, all of this without missing beat of the subject on hand. And again we all wondered if he would have major neck cramp for the next week. Nothing seemed to bother this extraordinary brilliant yet odd surgeon.

He would make an indelible impression on my hospital life as I had held him with high esteem, respect and wonderment, memories of these events lasting a lifetime.

Doctor Dettol, Flying Elements and Home Visiting G.P.

One of our esteemed G.P's, a General Practitioner-or Family Physician, was this middle-aged doctor, who was my Grandparents physician, and the man who would refer a major stream of patients to our consultant surgeon was Doctor Spencer Allyson. He had trained at Edinburgh University in the finest departments of medicine. So I determined the University must have stressed mightily upon him the immensity of how antiseptics and their use prevented most of mankind's diseases. Therefore a high level of dosing everything in sight with Dettol, that antiseptic which was used in many homes as-well-as the stronger preparation used in hospital wards, clinics and doctor's surgeries. Our Doctor Spencer Allyson was highly proficient at dosing everything in his world. Everything! The door to his surgery waiting room gave everyone a first indication that the world beyond it was probably swimming in Dettol since one's nose was accosted with 'extra strength' Dettol' when opening the door to his surgery. It was before the arrival of his first patient everyday that his cleaning lady would Dettol'ize everything.

33

She soaked the doorknobs, chairs, the hand bell, telephone, and pens pencils and of course, the glass thermometers as well as his beloved stethoscope and reflex hammer.

Should his patients have a cough and a cold they were 'instructed' to look away from the doctor, or if they were going to cough to actually stand up and cough to wards the far corner of the room! Under no circumstances was our 'Dettol Doctor' going to be directly exposed to those invisible invaders those unseen Flying *Elements*, those germs of myriad diseases.

This physician, to his mind, was a bastion, a Fortress of hygiene. When asked any question regarding any aspect of a patient's health or when a nurse might want to clarify an order he had given, he would always begin In his finely attuned Scottish accent, "Actually, as you may know, contra-indicated in this arena of this disease process, one could expect a variety of outcomes." This answer, uttered as eloquently and precise as the bard's greatest poetic accomplishment, was in response to *any question*. It seemed amazing, to we lesser souls, we had no idea what he meant, the words perhaps dramatically spoken with great diction and fine elocution, never seemed to answer anyone's question. So we asked again and hoped for a more simple reply. The answers never actually came; his mind was racing on to search the annals of medicine or how he could combat those 'flying elements' of invaders and bugs.

Doctor Spencer Allyson was a good man. His aging patients loved him. Actually he had very few patients under 39 years old. I always theorized that once the younger patients experienced his rather odd behavior they found a different family doctor. Doctor Allyson was one of the dying breed of physicians, he made House Calls morning or evening depending upon the severity of the patient. He had Dettol and so he was unafraid! His surgery patients, lining up in the darkened waiting room were generally seen in the morning so that after lunch each day he climbed into his spotless antique Rover car and made his home visits. These visits could probably have been done much faster but he had to follow his very delicate protocol, where again, Dettol ruled and swabs accumulated.

On arriving at the patients home and getting out of his car he always patted his bulging jacket pockets, one on each side. The jacket, which didn't match his pants, was one of those large loosely hanging corduroy sports jackets with leather elbow patches and a leather backed collar. Just as a surgeon would don the long green operating room gown, our Doctor Allyson's corduroy jacket was his own operating gown-for all events, emergencies or otherwise.

In the left hand pocket were clean cotton wool balls, lots of them. In the two inside pockets were two bottles of Dettol and the outside right hand pocket was for the wet Dettol swabs! No bugs lived in that jacket, but it did have its strong recognizable fragrance, everyone could smell his Dettol before you could see him!

He would approach a patient's home, and in those days most of the houses had either substantial brass doorknockers or bell-pulls'. The bell-pulls' handle, where you would find a bell pull knob, and when pulled, a ring of bells in the kitchen occurred to announce someone at the front door. Our germ free doctor would first try not touch the door knob handle but wait until the occupants opened the door from inside, therefore, of course he would not need to use Dettol swabs on the door knob, and so remain free of any contact with possible pathogens!

There were times when he did have to go through the procedure of taking out of his pocket a clean, dry swab, then pouring Dettol over the swab to thoroughly sanitize the bell pull knob. Once swabbed, the now dirty, still wet swab would be transferred into the *dirty* pocket.

Upon being led upstairs to his sick patients' bedroom, he never failed to ask his series of questions, their main complaint? How long? Where is the pain? Did you vomit? How are your bowels? Do you feel feverish? Are you dizzy or have a headache'? This was the same sequence of questions for his entire list of patients, which gave Doctor Allyson a foundational direction towards a diagnosis. I believe all his patients knew the questions my heart from previous encounters and were ready for him.

Doctor Allyson either had very poor hearing or alternatively his hearing ability was brilliant. After cleaning both the earpieces over and over, then the bell or chest piece with the same usual routine of smothering in Dettol. Stethoscope, once clean and packed into his ears he would place the chest piece carefully, methodically on each side of the patient's back, going from the top to bottom, then, similarly listen to the front of the chest. Once all the breathing 'in and out' was complete, he wanted silence. He wanted complete silence from the patient and anyone else in the room whilst he carefully moved the chest piece over the heart where he could determine a cardiac rhythm and its irregularities. I believe he knew his heart sounds and their QRS complex quite well.

That stethoscope was his medical investigatory tool, rather than to wait for a laboratory or x-ray study which were at the end of a long waiting line. He was equally adept at listening to a cacophony of bowel sounds, a symphony of slow or rapid rumblings of a healthy bowel or perhaps a bowel in distress and there would begin a new realm of investigation, perhaps poking and applying pressure with his fingers or hands pushing downwards, or even supporting one side of the abdomen, whilst pushing then releasing with the other hand on the opposite side.

He might exclaim during these physical explorations, that "No, McBurneys point is quite clear", referring to the abdominal area midway between the crest of the right hip across to the umbilicus, the point under which lies the Appendix. If Appendicitis were present the patient would howl with the increased pain, "*Ahaa, an Inflammatory Appendix*", he would remark with great certainty!

Doctor Spencer Allyson was well read, and he loved medical history. However, it seemed somewhat of a dichotomy when trying to put his idea of 'Dowsing with Dettol' everything he touched. This was, in essence, to kill the germs that caused diseases. But he was no fan of Louis Pasteur whom he believed to be a chemist of no greater distinction than his plagiarism of his fellow Frenchman Antoine Bechamp. It was Bechamp, who had published lots of verified scientific articles on disease causation, and it was Bechamp that was the true investigator and scientist for he was a biologist, doctor, chemist and a physicist, and it was he, Bechamp that had discovered the existence of microbes. He had done this research to identify microbes, the Germ Theory, and had discovered the minutest living particulate matter, the microzymas and their unique characteristics. He had clearly proved that disease, its origin, was within the body and hence, our own level of well being-our health was the true determinant for our recovery and longevity.

It was apparently proved later, that chemist Pasteur fraudulently published *his* findings creating a totally opposite conclusion! Before the truth was evident, Pasteur became a hero, a monument to this *germ theory* that the pharmaceutical industry began creating a plethora of drugs to combat the bugs.

So our Doctor Allyson loved his Dettol and praised the 'real germs' that were our 'friendly bugs' like those Bacillus coli whose remarkable ability to decompose carbohydrates by the formation of acid in our intestines. And so, as always when he gave his brief lectures on immunity or infections we learned of rogues and real hero's of modern medicine, as well as the disinfecting fragrance that emanated from the last Dettol swab hiding in a far corner of his jacket pocket to stop the spread of those bad bugs and flying elements!

CHAPTER 2

Medical Ward

The Power of Ireland and India in our Midst.

The Medical Ward was on the furthest wing to the east of the Fortress building, an addition to the much older building which seemed totally out of style with the other patient buildings. To get there, visitors and staff had to go through the main long hospital corridor, then after going through noisily clanging double doors at the end of the corridor, a narrow tunnel opened onto the patio-like veranda. Then for eighty yards or so with only a sparse patio cover for shelter, it was open to the weather come rain, snow or occasional sunshine. So, the get back from the Medical Ward to the main dining room, administration, x-ray or laboratory and all the other Wards this gauntlet of hostile weather had to be dealt with. If patients were on a stretcher, wheelchair or they were slow moving invalids balancing life and limb with a walking stick their race was on! So was the wind.

When I, or other Student Nurses, were taking patients across this veranda especially in blustery winds on wet and cold days, I would tell the patients they were blessed since they did not have to endure more of this brief outdoor sojourn like the patients in our regional Tuberculosis Hospital. These patients were rolled out of their rooms each day onto their extended patios in sunshine or in snow. Breathing clean, fresh air so invigorating, that healing touch from the wind, so therapeutic and it sounded like a great story!

On our medical floor, a different kind of drama was always playing out. Different and stern faced, thin as a rake, was the Medical Ward's Lady in Navy Blue, this was Anne Janiceton, with her powerful high pitched squeaky voice.

Her uniform was more starched, sharper edged, had more razor like edges than any other of the Sisters, the Ladies in Navy Blue or the meticulous Student Nurses and their uniforms. In some misty vision of the past she had been married to a plumber who had become a local councilman, and apparently after two years on the City Council and after many late evening meetings, he had engaged in a noisy, robust verbal fisty-cuffs against an opposing councilman after which he up and died on the council chamber floor in full view of councilmen, the interested public and a couple of local newspaper reporters. A grand finale to his probable legislative career on the council. The tragic story was given front-page news for the weekly Saturday Edition, all of which may have left Anne Janiceton, a highly-strung and nervous widow.

A photo of him in a black suit, a black a tie and lovely, well polished black shoes standing proudly looking out to sea on Blackpool's wet sandy beach, adorned one corner of her mighty desk, a memory of a legislative life cut short. Neither I nor anyone else, every heard her speak of him, perhaps too sad a story.

Anne Janiceton was Irish from the lovely town of Cork, but there was only a whisper of her Irish accent in her voice, but her short fuse, to a full-blown temper was always a breath away. Any wrong action of a Student Nurse created an explosion of the best of Irish expressions of exasperations and fury. Comedians and other literary men of tragedies would have benefitted from her outbursts! Only on St. Patrick's Day did we notice a cession of hostilities, but alas that was only once a year.

Her desk was almost always far too tidy, everything lined up with everything else, if anything was on the desk only a meticulous fraction of an inch separated one pile of papers from another, for her *everything* must be in perfect order, the patients charts likewise in perfect continuity.

As a Student Nurse in this arena of authority and precision, for me, was my daily adversary; she inspected everything the Student Nurses did. It did not matter whether a brand new Student Nurse, or one ready to graduate after three grueling years. It was not a happy rotation to get the Medical Ward for three months each year of our student days. The greatest joy on this Ward was working the night shift and being in-charge, if verbal storms were to come they would be at the end of our shift-and we could be spared that ear-bending assault if there was a major patient incident that happened where we had resolved the issue. As always at the end of our training we were much better prepared for what was ahead. What I learned there was part of the sure foundation of all of my days in every aspect of nursing and the excellent quality nursing care that I gave. So my regards for teaching me so well, I salute her.

The daily parade began at 9 am precisely, it was a sight to behold; it was a parade of personalities, of colorful uniforms, of chart and notes, of tension and high anxiety, these Grand Rounds were militaristic in purpose and execution. They occurred on each Ward, but at different times.

The parade began with one of our two Internal Medicine Consultants, each highly respected, each an excellent diagnostician and authoritarian; they were in command, indeed, whilst I trained there Sister Janiceton, and these two Consultants wielded great power, they spoke-we obeyed!

It was customary for the Consultant to stop briefly at the door to sister's office to ask, "How is the morning going?" then stride down the corridor first to the Male Ward, and when finished there, to the Female Ward.

Since all the patients had already been washed bathed, shaved, had clean sheets they were now presentable. Patient's pressure areas had been washed with soap and water dried then methylated spirits rubbed vigorously over buttocks, heels and elbows then dusted with talcum powder. This ritual kept bedsores away, and it worked and the patients even smelled nice for these Grand Rounds!

This done, the beds had all been lined up to the 'line' created by the wooden floor boards down the length of the Ward, in military fashion down on that marker. The patients for the most part were made to lie still, propped up on two or three pillows, their brown counterpane's folded precisely to at a point of 28" from the head of the bed, so if you were to look at the beds from the Wards entrance, then on each side of the Ward the 12 to 14 beds and their occupants lined up like they were on parade, but no one saluted.

These patients, expectant of great pronouncements from our Internal Medicine Consultant about their condition and a hopeful recovery were told not to talk, cough or be noisy in any way. Sister Janiceton, had already warned all her male patients that there would be 'no passing of wind or farting, no vulgar burping, or talking' and they clearly got the message. When I first saw this parade I almost expected the patients to raise up and salute en masse to this mighty General, this pillar of medical knowledge. It never happened alas, the saluting that is or jumping to attention, but what did happen on one blustery, wet and windy morning with rain clattering on the windows, was funny. An older repeat patient let go with a mighty, explosive fart. It was loud and long, and everybody in that parade grinned sheepishly. The anxious patient was always complaining of 'abdominal troubles', and so he proved it!

Our Consultant on that day was Doctor Paul Richard Justin, brilliant as always, but generally stony faced bellowed across the Ward, *"Catch that noisy, onerous fellow before he gets out"*! Everybody that was awake and alert enough laughed and applauded, I too was delighted with the response! Such was the unexpected humour for that day, proving he was human after all!

The normally quiet parade consisted of Doctor Justin or his colleague Doctor Trevor Potter depending on who had been 'on call' the night before, then came the Sister Janiceton, carrying patient charts, followed by her two Staff Nurses, looking so prim and proper. The House Physician, Doctor Nimesh Patel, followed with his Senior Intern Doctor Randy Davidson (an intern newly graduated), both were usually unshaven and unkempt especially after an active 'life saving' night on the Wards.

Behind them came the Dietician, an overweight buxom lady who seemed to know exactly what foods should be eaten for each diagnosis, remarkable in those long ago days. She liked to share her information with this retinue of medical and nursing specialization, but her monotone voice would have us all dozing off by the end of her first paragraph of nutritious wisdom. Doctor Justin frequently would cut her off after she had answered his first couple of questions of, 'How well the patient was eating?' or 'Did the food make them vomit?' and 'Did it appear that there may be any allergies related to the diet?' In response our buxom lass would answer in barely a whisper.

Following the Dietician came the Adonis of the parade, the Physiotherapist. He was as bald as a bean, too early for his 31 years but brawny, muscular and always somewhat suntanned. This in itself seem highly incredulous, because how on earth could this atlas of a man find enough English sun even in the summer, never mind the snow or darkened and windy, cloud laden sky. Our windswept northern English autumn, winter and well into spring days, it was hard to find enough sunshine to even look into the heavens in search of this golden globe! 'No' all the nurses decided that his suntanned look came from some French exotic crème that he sent to Paris to obtain. We again wildly conjured up was that he had invented a reflecting mirror that surrounded his body completely and when a sliver of sunlight flashed by the sun rays would somehow change his pale skin to this golden, award winning sun tan. His first name was Brendan but for some reason he would never tell us his last name, and when asked, he would just shrug his massive shoulders in the '*I don't want to tell you*' way and said nothing.

I always enjoyed being part of these Grand Rounds, it felt like this was an extension of some renowned University with its mighty Medical teaching staff, it was inspiring!

Physiotherapist Brendan's daily routine never varied and he arrived on the Wards at the exact time each day. On the Medical Ward he made sure all the respiratory diagnosed patients were doing breathing exercises exactly as he instructed; on the Orthopedic Ward he pulled and pushed and stretched limbs until they ached. On surgical floor, he got patients out of bed and walked them, balanced them and to those who had surgery the previous day he brought pain and anguish to this handful of newly scarred surgical patients as he hauled them to the 'right' position with lovely threats that he would be back tomorrow for the real exercise.

Those patients hated him, well almost, as they sneered behind his back when he left the Ward.

On the Obstetrics and Gynecological Wards Hugh did his rounds demanding abdominal exercises, deep breathing and least to have legs dangled out of bed. Yes, we student's and our patient's all knew him with his 'torture routines'. However, his private life we knew little about, only that on the wall behind his simple do-it-yourself desk in his small office I did see a black and white photo of himself with a stunning, lovely Caribbean beauty, his wife I thought, and a little boy of five or six, who looked a lot like him but had the colour of his light skinned Jamaican mother, the photo was obliviously taken on a bright sunny day under a palm tree on a beach close to the ocean. Under the picture in small print was the title, *'In Jamaica, our home in the sun in 1954'*. Another secret waiting to be told.

In the parade of the Grand Rounds behind Brendan, our came the 'Recreations' lady, she was there to answer possible questions about a patient's interest or involvement in any of the crafts or books that she carried. The answer she gave would indicate that the patient's mental status was improving, was still intact or alternatively perhaps, a lack of interest indicating depression or worse. On her seemingly old and over-burdened cart came magazines, books, newspapers, jigsaw puzzles and crafts of all descriptions.

The Student Nurses perhaps unkindly but actually in a warmer friendly way called our Recreations lady, simply 'Nikki'. Her actual name was Nicola Prentice the kind of name that old Barrack Room Ballard's are written in prose and sang melodiously about. The 'Nikki' title came both from her lovely name and recreational-hospital skills, and with that huge dark brown cart she laboriously pushed from Ward to Ward and down the Fortress's long corridors, over the open-air verandas. Everyone knew she was coming because the wheels of her cart squealed and screeched, wheels that had probably travel many hundreds of miles upon the hospital corridors without even a single drop of oil. Occasionally she would accidentally hit the corner of some wall or doorway and indelibly leave a dark indentation from one corner or another of her lumbering, heavy and well-laden cart.

44

We all loved her, she always seemed joyful, always had a radiant smile for everyone, even those more miserable patients scowling at her who wanted nothing from her. She had a job to do and she did it with radiance, if you met her coming along some stretch of corridor she would more likely than not, be singing quietly to herself that lovely old hymn, Amazing Grace.

Joining the parade now came the Social Worker, a very thin and very tall—perhaps 6'2" lady with long straight blond hair simply flowing over her angular shoulders. She was pretty for her age, I guessed in her thirties, (everybody over thirty was old according to our eighteen year old generation). She had all the Male Nurses thinking of her as a stunner, a real beauty. As a group we were probably just over half her age; so in this instance, we ignored that rule. Probably all the lads felt very masculine when she, it seemed, purposely smiled at us for a period of seconds that seemingly extended far too long, it was almost a 'come hither' look, our interpretation, of course. None of us ever, I think, got close to her, but our translated implied look of hers-to us, had its lovely fleeting moments.

This tall lovely lass, her name was Dahlia Forester, must have been educated in the shadowy secret underground bastion of MI5. That super secret service organization where she could get any and all information about anyone at a moment notice, and would appear quite nonchalant as if she always knew it; a mysterious woman of beauty and talent.

She was at the top of her profession. She knew each patient diagnosis, length of time expected to be bed ridden in hospital, or at home. She knew many family members were at home to help the discharged patient, as well as what profession or job and how the employer paid the benefits. She knew the fine print of Socialized Medicine and how it impacted patient, hospital and physician. Dahlia was good, *really good.* Her mind must have had multitudinous convolutions to store the information she hid about so many patients. Her office, which she shared with another social worker, who dealt only with the Mental Hospital and whose files were meticulously ordered. However, Dahlia's side of the office was strewn everywhere with papers, files, hand written notes pinned by tacks to the wall, medical magazines, newspapers from many yesterday's, and a grand collection of walking sticks and old, well-used wooden crutches. Two small bulletin boards were smothered in coloured paper notes held on by tacks- and there were lots of tacks. Her two wooden clumsy, two drawer filing cabinets, one on top of the other were piled high with charts, and charts coming out of the drawers because they were crammed in too tightly, from patients discharged recently, I surmised after seeing them.

She did have a telephone on her desk, but it was quite cleverly surrounded on three sides by the most recent patient's charts, which needed further clarification, and a stack of Social Service forms.

I think all the Nurses, Male and Female, first year or third year held her in wonderment that she could be so good at what she did, since being part of the morning parade' (for her on each Ward at different times) could spend so much time in these parades. She would also meet directly with patients, their relatives, or occasionally one-on-one meetings with doctors to discuss patient issues, and then to go back to her office to do her own charting, and telephone communications. Dahlia had the knack of being at peace with all of this, seemingly enjoying her major role there.

At the end of this morning parade, a retinue of great minds and thinkers were the Medical Students, one or two senior year medical students. These students more often than not were male, but occasionally there was a female medical student all generally coming from fairly well off families. For the general working class of Britain there was little chance to get into university and then take 5 or 6 years of intense study-without the security of family finances. But there was the rare occasional working class family youth who was academically brilliant and so was pushed and supported by their teachers and headmaster to apply for whatever scholastic grants would be available, and once pursed and gained then the rite of passage into university, then medical school opened up a new life, a new world.

This also accounted for the difference in speech of the wealthy families' children who spoke a more refined or cultured English whereas the families of the working class children spoke with their very pronounced Lancastrian, Yorkshire, and Brummie or Gordie dialect. These students fortunate to get financial grants most of the way through to their final Medical Degree would move into a world of more finer worldly living than that of their parents. These achievers with their strong accents and dialects generally could weave between 'refined diction and elocution' back into their local dialects, we admired them and would do anything extra for them.

The long line of professional families who had sent their children to universities and hence continued to have abundant finances would produce physicians who were not 'in it' for the monetary reward. Generally all had that sense of becoming a doctor to heal, and cure, and discover the way to a new drug or a better operative procedure. Their lives then, were dedicated to *saving mankind* rather than to gain greater earthly riches. Perhaps this was a spiritual goal, for a 'greater human goodness, and even godliness'. Attributes that helped to create varying degrees of eccentricity, and it seemed that when eccentricity became a major characteristic in their life, that was when both amazement, puzzlement and humour was generated for the onlooker, observer and casual passer-by who would either smile and quietly approve or disdainfully frown and look down upon our troupe of 'bizarre medical and mad eccentrics'.

I watched them in action before my very eyes. I saw first hand, and listened to so many conversations that compendiums of great memories were created. These Eccentrics lived in a different world and yet seemed always incredibly brilliant at whatever specialty they claimed as theirs.

At the very back of this parade with the medical students came the third year 'we know it all' Student Nurses, and each Ward had one or two of these third years nurses, this gave the Grand Rounds parade a total of twelve to fifteen characters as they marched then stopped, and marched again at each bedside.

There was always strict disciple and certainly 'no talking' between any one whilst the Consultant, our majestic man held court. Looks between companions on these marches were the only accepted means of communication. In a way it was both quite serious and quite humorous, smiling or laughing politely when the Chief asked one of the patients a 'yes' or 'no' question but got a story of high drama, where eventually the Consultant would have to stop the patient, then repeat the question which would eventually lead to the answer. If allowed to keep speaking the patients could tell their life stories!

Always the physicians had to have a good deal of patience when asking questions, and they became so adept at interrupting the older generation of patients as they wove their intricate story from a simple question, perhaps, why they had a cough, or perhaps when they first felt the pain.

These older folks, after being asked a simple question, never gave a simple answer, but instead provided a detailed account of some event, I had intimate knowledge about this dilemma. My own Mum had that story telling gift of attempting to answer our family doctors simple question of, "_How long ago was it_ when you noticed the headache at the front of your head?" Her reply would begin by remembering, and so telling the doctor of how she was able to get in at their usual boarding house for the holiday week, so since they had to wait for their room to be ready, they had gone to the North Shore of Blackpool, their holiday town, to a friend of their neighbor who had recommended both the good companionship, and the good food of the boarding house. They had got to the boarding house early in the day, but couldn't get into their bedroom till later in that day, so they decided to go for a brisk walk down the promenade. It was just before the tide was fully in, and so, ...the story could go on, and on. If the doctor didn't stop the story by again repeating the key question of 'exactly how long ago_was it when the pain began?'

Those physicians more skilled at intervening to stop the rambling story, or were far too busy to let the patient keep going, would almost seem impatient or bad mannered and so got the answers to their History's and Physicals or other investigations more rapidly than others doctors.

It was these patient responses of great stories still untold that the consultant would perhaps slap his hands together, or twist his mustache, or drop his chin down to his chest then slumping his shoulders, those significant non-verbal communications did their duty.

But invariably the doctor would cut off the story sometimes with a clever or funny quip that would stop the patient and have all of us in the entourage laugh or smile approvingly.

If a patient was a repeat 'Pulmonary Lunger' of which the Medical Ward had many, these less fortunate patients who had succumbed to the damp, soot laden air and where their lungs were no longer able to facilitate enough oxygen to keep both their brain and whole body energized with life giving breath.

These respiratory compromised patients seemed to be always in a state of spluttering, coughing, wheezing and occasionally spitting up a massive glob of greenish phlegm. Their faces too were a purple-red and when they coughed their paroxysm of strained respirations just to get another breath, another moment of life—their faces became that beetroot deep red colour with their facial veins more pronounced and ready to explode at any moment! These men were part of our 'Wheezing Old Geezers', for Geriatrics had many of them too.

These patients, propped up on five or six pillows, probably dreaded the daily question asked by our Consultant's, and what must have appeared to these patients looking at the entourage now at their bedside, and remembering the less than gentle instructions given to all patients by the Ward Sister not to speak or make any unruly noise whilst the Doctor-Mr. Justin made his rounds. Hence, either the desire or the need to cough, or the face to face questioning from this learned fellow would generate only a whispered answer or would create a further bout of strained coughing! Difficult for the patient, but I do clearly remember taking several extra deep breaths to help the patient over this difficulty, unconsciously driven yet remembering my earlier childhood of having sever Asthma attacks and struggling to breathe. They didn't help the patient, but I tried breathing deeply just in sympathy!

Occasionally there were younger patients, perhaps late teens and these patient's almost always generated some attempts at humour from the Chief. He may ask the teenager, "*What were you doing late last night*"? Or" *Did the police constable bring you in?*" or" "*Are you trying to get out of work?*"

These little quips may have been said to put the young man or woman with some ease, but they never got a smile from these young patients. However, the older professionals in the entourage laughed courteously for the doctors' benefit, not from the inappropriate joke. We, the Student Nurses, always thought these jokes were inappropriate and pathetic.

The Nurses at the rear of the parade really enjoyed this period of time. It meant no physical work during rounds, and apart from very quiet whispers to each other about what happened last night, or a brief discussion of the weekend's result of our local football team, and our advice on how they could have played better.

The Rounds were interesting and sometimes really enjoyable made even more so if there were disagreements between physicians on a choice of drug or the need for surgery, even raised voices, oh excitement! The refined accents of the Oxford or Cambridge educated physicians mingling with a clipped Indian voice with that distinctive pronunciation of each word, or perhaps the voice from a West Indian Resident with its almost lyrical musical tones. There was perhaps the voice of the Scottish Highlands or Lowlands with the softer Edinburgh University educated ladies or wee lassies. And there was never any doubt when we heard the softer gentler romantic voice of an Irishman or woman.

The morning Grand Rounds, this entourage, was probably going on in every hospital in Great Britain in much the same way. This was how the medical profession from the towers of authority and knowledge communicated to their staff and to these hospitalized patients. The consultant sharing modes of therapy whilst his residents and housemen, might seek advice on a course of medication, further surgery or other modes of therapy.

Grand Rounds on Medical Ward and elsewhere, were within themselves an Institution unto behold!

On the Medical Ward there was always much to see and do and learn.

There was the common treatment for Congestive Heart Failure, a Kidney Disease, or a Venous or Lymphatic Disease where draining the grossly edematous swollen legs with large bore needles. These needles, totally different from the Intramuscular needles, looked like a Lance from some Knight in Shining Armor. These needle 'lances' had several holes around its sturdy shaft of 3 inches, which were placed into the lower legs as the patient was in a Fowlers Position-sitting upright in bed with each leg dangling over the side of the bed with feet supported. These well placed needles effectively and slowly drained away the body's excessive and overloaded circulatory fluids. This fluid, the body's lymph, had been 'pushed' into the cellular spaces of the body causing the swelling, and since water finds the lowest part of the body in this case, the ankles, legs and frequently lower back, which would then becomes edematous. This is where anyone could press their fingers into the skin and make 'indentations', finger marks, were the skin would not spring back to its normal shape, hence oedema and most likely the culprit was Congested Heart Failure.

On Medical Ward as elsewhere were the fascinating voices of the physicians from India, and I think all the male nurses did their best to mimic their voices. We had grown up with dear old Peter Sellars on the Goon Show who had, it seemed, perfected the Indian speech mannerisms and we all had learned from him earlier in our lives how to speak '*Indian*'.

As a prank, especially on night shift, I and the other male nurses frequently played telephone games on the female nurses on other Wards. We would pretend to be a new Resident or Houseman giving innocuous orders to these unsuspecting Student Nurse who answered the phone. In our very best impersonated Indian voices we would give an urgent order for a newly invented drug. It worked more often than not and caused some of the nurses to become very angry with us when they discovered our deception.

On the Medical Ward, and occasionally on Geriatrics we had a delightful 'protem' Resident, he was Indian, and after coming to know him I would hire him in a minute. This was Doctor Dinesh Malhotra and he was specializing in internal medicine with a particular emphasis in cardiology. He had begun his long trek to our Fortress hospital in the cold north of England from the second most populous country in the world, 'Bharat' he would tell me, which is the Hindi word of 'India'. He came from Mysore a state in Southern India but went to Medical School and completed his Internship in

New Delhi. Whilst there, and completing his love for India's Punjabi, Gujarati and Urdu languages, but in the midst of taking an acting role in a film he was notified by his sister Deepika also a doctor, doing a residency in pediatrics at the well respected hospital great Ormond Street Hospital in Bloomsbury, London. She had learned of a position for a 'protem' position at our hospital group and so Doctor Dinesh landed at our Fortress Hospital. He was bright and had a great memory as many Indian physicians seemed to have, but for me most of all he was funny and a great conversationalist I first met him on one of my night shifts on the medical Ward, I had asked him to pronounce one of the patients who had just died, it was one of the patients where I had been immediately aware of his heart stopping as I held his radial pulse. Quickly checking his Carotid pulses and finding nothing, then checked his pupils, which were unreactive and he had stopped breathing, I ran to the medicine cabinet, got a 20 cc glass syringe, spinal needle and glass vial of Coramine broke the glass top and drew in the 10cc ran back to his bedside opened up his pajama jacket, found the space between the ribs, and *plunged the spinal needle into his heart*, drew up blood for assurance it was in the heart, then pushed the Coramine into his heart, withdrawing the needle I then pounded his chest vigorously to shock it, finally using the heel of my hand to massage the chest area over the heart. This frantic, yet hopeful way to stimulate the heart into a living rhythm again. Too primitive, perhaps, but what else was there? Didn't work, but the effort was always heroic. Well, I thought so and always tried. Doctor Malhotra arrived at the bedside half an hour later, asked for the diagnosis or probable diagnosis from the chart, if patient had cried out and what were my interventions. This was a rare question; usually the physicians quickly pronounced the patient and generally left the Ward. However, this simple question, an element of his curiosity, immediately created a bond between us. Doctor Malhotra was a wealth of information, I would guess he was eight or nine years older than I, but we seemed to get on really well together. I did on one occasion, perhaps in bad taste, tried my best Peter Sellars Indian accent, *"Oh, goodness gracious me"* I said, but Doctor Malhorta smiled broadly and said " You need more practice". *"How about some lovely chapatti and chips"* he replied and spoken in his more well pronounced Indian-English accent, saying again, "Now you have another line to pronounce like an Indian." A man of good humour! On another late night shift I was quite surprised to see Doctor Dinesh Malhorta, stop by the Ward for a cup of our salted coffee, and again he was in a chatty mood. So I took this unique opportunity to ask him a ton of questions about his homeland and its customs. We got our coffee and sat at the Ward's central night table. He struck me as a handsome man and he would probably be a 'good catch' for some deserving Nurse. So emboldened I asked him if he was married or engaged, he wore no rings and was approaching 30 years of age so this was a good question, I thought. He said his parents had betrothed him to Bipasha Khapadia, a girl four years younger than he, when he was just eleven years. Since, I was genuinely surprised by this old Indian custom, he explained that both parents were careful in whom they chose for future partners for their children, as they used familiarity with each other's families and backgrounds. They tried to use a perceived future prospect for their children based on position in life, business, or religious beliefs, and the all-important achievement of parents and their family backgrounds. The families' decisions were careful, loving and wise. It was a custom done for Indian families for many generations and in the vast majority, this childhood 'promise of marriage' of their sons and daughters worked well, and Dinesh finished by telling me he was to be married one year from now at home in Mysore, and all was well, even though he had not seen Bipasha for almost five years. I was puzzled, impressed and happy for him all at once. "You are a good man Doctor Dinesh Malhotra, I'm excited for you, your wife to be, and your success", I said. That late and interesting chat well into the night, almost uninterrupted by patients asking for pain medicine, or assistance getting out of, or into bed, I found this proud Indian gentleman Physician fascinating. He told me of India's 22 official languages and its more than 350 dialects, he told me of India's Independence Day, on August 15th and that the National Anthem song was called 'Jana Gana Mana'; and a National song going back to 1896 was 'Vande Mataram, which he then tried to sing the first few lines, but gave up because he was out of rhythm, chord and melody. I learned of the national symbols of India and what they meant, the

Bird, Peacock being sacred, beautiful, mystical and graceful, and the Lotus Flower, and the Tiger, Lord of the Jungle with its power, yet majestic and full of Royalty. The Banyan tree, a gathering place for all Indian's, including the myriad of creatures that lived in and around the tree, symbolic of a place to meet and greet. Doctor Malhotra was most particularly proud of an athletic event that the world looked at with admiration and praise. It was not a major Cricket event as I was beginning to suspect for he loved Cricket and the battle for the 'Ashes', but an event that stamped national pride in India, Nepal and in England all at the same time. It was the event of May 29, 1953 that caught, the world's imagination it was the planting of three flags at top of the world's highest mountain Mount Everest it was that national flag of India, design adopted only 6 years earlier in 1947, the flags of Nepal, with the Union Jack of Great Britain, were also planted on top this intensely cold, windy and snow capped mighty peak. The human spirit, forever is forging on and up, into unknown territory and conquering it. This was truly a great accomplishment, it was teamwork finely tuned, and it was true athleticism, the aspect of physical endurance to succeed. Remarkable in this singular accomplishment of man, the conquering of Mount Everest by Sir Edmund Hilary and his team of climbers, and the support team that kept the mountainous camps supplied during that momentous climb. Another hospital physician who held this historic event in high regard even to the point of having the photo on the wall of the corridor leading to his office, Doctor Edward Potter our Gerontologist, hopefully at some point the two Physicians would meet and enjoy the shared admiration of the Everest Climb. If they didn't meet, I'd share to each one separately to other's Mount Everest appreciation.

I met Doctor Dinesh Malhotra many more times, usually at patient's bedside over the year he was there, and those meetings were always respectfully friendly. The weekend before he was gone for good, he brought over for me a beautifully coloured decal of the Indian flag held on a rope, and at each end of the rope which was held in the mouth of a Tiger on one end and on the other end held in the mouth of an Elephant. I had no 'gift' for him, but enthusiastically wished his marriage to his childhood betrothed, Bipasha to be Happy, Healthy and Fruitful.

Chapter 3

Operating Room

Open Bellies, Squirting Vessels and Ancient Instruments

The 'OR' home of imaginary instruments of torture, pleasure, fear, horror, the macabre, and ancient mysterious medieval dungeon like weapons, each frightening and each having its own unique characteristics. However, they were all important in their own design.

That glorious time in OR when it came to the assignment of the operating room. It was the department of cloak and dagger with everyone wearing huge facemasks. It was even a mystery of sorts, where patients came in for one reason for an operation, and left having a different operation. This was the world of blood and guts where the 'theatre' of the 'OR' was dressed in green. Green walls, green gowns that tied at the neck and almost touched the floor, green caps that always seemed too big, green cloth face masks that left only the tiniest slit of face-for your eyes and the ever present green surgical towels for covering tables, trays, surgical instruments, and other equipment. There were huge green sterile towels made with holes in the middle or with elongated slits and green towels made like large individuals men's pant legs-used when a patient, under anesthesia had their legs held up on stirrups so the surgeon or gynecologist had access to a 'waiting' posterior! The only white colour came from white Wellington Boots that everyone wore and the white floor tiles.

Our operating room had fairly quick access towards the end of the hospital's long corridor for the obstetrics, labor and delivery Wards and the huge gynecological Ward. However, for the surgery and orthopedic Wards, patients on their stretchers had to be wheeled down the long, unevenly green tiled corridor. Its poor lighting cast a rather ominous glow that never quite reached into darker recesses of doorways or smaller hallways leading off to left or right of the corridor.

The well-worn tile of this cavernous corridor echoed footfalls, voices and trolleys clanging, noises from people, carts and stretchers. Through the darkness, when only the night shift staff walked with purpose through this gauntlet of an unending passage, the sounds became even more exaggerated and the echoing voices, seemed more guarded. Occasionally a lone stretcher plying its way to the operating room had an eerie muffled character all of its own, with screeches occasionally of unoiled wheels with quiet yet odd whispered voices and anxious, perhaps tearful questions from the fearful patient asking about his or her survival.

The entrance to the Operating Room, which faced down this endless corridor, had a huge double doorway. Its larger than life floor to ceiling doors were made of heavy black rubber and the frame of the doors on each side had been gouged, bent and scarred by the corners of the sturdy metal trolleys (stretches) as they were pushed on through into the operating room.

The huge Operating Room black rubber doors showed only a minimum of wear with a slight concave indentation, even after hundreds upon hundreds of trolleys had hit the same general area on their way into the bowels of the operating room.

The two huge heavy black rubber doors into the operating room were clearly, very clearly marked in large unmistakable white letters *In* and *Out* and to add to this simple message, below both In and Out were the red lettering on white background the words *No Smoking*. The English language, elegant in its simplicity on these particular doors held but two words in opposition to each other

In and Out; the two other words an implicit, straight forward, an incontrovertible demand, *NO SMOKING!*

Easily understood by everyone else, these four precious words, *in, out, no smoking,* may well have been missing from the lexicon of Doctor David Peter Alexander, as we are about to discover.

Since there was no pre-op, or post-op recovery rooms, all the trolleys going in went through the obviously marked *IN* door; and so going out after surgery, the trolley would simply go out through the clearly marked *OUT* door. It was an easy, simple and uncomplicated, clearly marked route. During the night when no further operations were in progress, even the cleaners, custodians and other tech's went in and out through the correctly marked doors, it seemed so simple. It just didn't need a specialized degree to open the right door!

The marking on the doors was actually a critical characteristic for the interior of our operating room. A trolley bringing the patient IN, who would then be transferred onto the Operating Room table, so that the empty trolley was carefully wheeled around the head of the OR table and back out into the corridor through the OUT door. This carefully planned route was made so that the Anesthesiologist would not have to move his small cart, which contained all of his anesthesia needs, as needles, syringes, drugs in glass vials with their tiny metal files close at hand. It also contained various sized airways, intubation tubes, and face masks- those dome shaped basket-like metal sieves (that were equally well designed to drain water from vegetables), but had pads of cotton wool placed around the inside of this dome. This basin-like bowl was later placed over a patients face, and the anesthesiologist would slowly allow droplets of Chloroform onto the cotton wool which, when the vapor was inhaled, created that unconscious sleep, the tri-light zone of anesthesia.

On this cart in an upright position were the small metal and different coloured cylinders. Amongst them were Oxygen and Nitrous Oxide, their cylinder holders welded onto the side of this small cart that also had several drawers. In the first drawer attached to the underside of the top platform surface, were vials of drugs from Sodium Pentothal, central nervous system and other muscle relaxants, cardiac stimulants, Coramine, Adrenaline and anti-convulsive drugs. There were various needles from subcutaneous to the longer ominous-looking spinal needles, the length of these needles would have any normal person take an extra breath, but the bore, (hole size) seemed like they should be used for watering the garden, not to be plunged *carefully of course*, between the bony vertebrae of a waiting, curved back of the spine. Bandages, Elastoplast's (band aids), tourniquets, lengths of red rubber tubing, skin markers and pens.

The second drawer was well stocked with red rubber endotracheal tubes from the delicate sized pediatric tubes to the large adult tubes, which seemed big enough to keep an elephant oxygenated.

The House Anesthesiologist, our esteemed Doctor Dennis Holt, maintained this little cart. He was a lanky, tall thin man, in his mid forties, who was perhaps the quietest, most gently spoken of all of our physicians. He was easy to please, stocked his own cart from our operating room supply room both before the days' surgeries began and at the end of the day just to be prepared for any late night operation requiring anesthesia. He was meticulous, had everything in its correct order and was always dressed in his own laundered operating room attire, rather than using the hospital supplied clothing. However there were times when this quiet, retiring professional lost complete and total control of his demeanor! His pale white face became engorged with a massive push of blood under an incredible and instantaneous hypertensive blood pressure rush that seemed it would send blood spurting out of his nostrils! Perhaps, even his once lily white ears, bursting now with bright beacon red blood throbbing ear lobes that any second would simply pop and send a spray of blood in all directions of the OR.

This apoplectic show was quite majestic, even a magical instant change from mild, quiet concentrated calculations of anesthesia to a man *possessed by a violent erupting rage*, where his language skills became unintelligible!

Our high voltage drama was not a singular episode, it happened with rather frightening regularity. I assumed, on seeing this for the first time, that with each cataclysmic event his blood pressure would force all four chambers of his heart to rupture in sequence and thereby give the recording examining pathologist a precise diagnosis for the cause of death as *'Heart Eruption and Failure'*. Precision indeed, these seemingly remarkable events occurred when our illustrious Surgical Consultant David Peter Alexander, had completed both his surgical Grand Rounds and his usual mid morning lecture, to whichever group of nurses that had eagerly awaited him. Well, now he was free to drop into the OR and check on his surgical Senior Houseman and observe progress or to suggest an alternative procedure.

If a particularly difficult, interesting or even if a surgery would require two surgeons, as an Abdominal Perineal Resection would require. So he would schedule the surgery to coincide with his timetable, and his Houseman would begin the surgery and *open* the abdomen cutting down into the peritoneal cavity, placing the retractors to be ready for his Consultant. Doctor Alexander would pop into the operating room to either instruct the Houseman or suggest an alternative operative procedure or realizing the surgery required two surgeons, he would go to the changing room and don the operating attire. However, when he knew he was there *only* to check on progress, offer advice or to simply to be available then his entrance into the OR was the creation of those *cataclysmic events*.

Doctor Alexander, who may have been a great lover of the written poetic word, would take any reading material he could get his hands on from either the male or female changing rooms. It didn't seem to matter whether it was financial page of a newspaper or *Woman's Own* magazine. Off he would go and sit on the 'pot', the toilet, reading these gems of information. There he would read and smoke. To be alone and silent in his thoughts perhaps, practicing how to define exquisite English terminology and observe or comprehend a spectacularly simple command on the OR Doors, but seemed outside of his vision and understanding.

Doctor David Peter with his half smoked cigarette magically glued to his upper left lip and just as miraculous was the ash of that cigarette hanging on to the remaining half, just tiny flakes of ash drifting downwards as another breath of inhaled smoked filled his waiting lungs. He was completely oblivious to the fact cigarette smoking cannot be done simply *everywhere*! Now, with smoke pouring out of his nostrils he would go *into* the Operating Room through the *OUT* door. A major error of unintended consequences! We thought, or was it?

Behind that Out door, now swinging inwards with its own heavy rubberized weight, slamming into the chair and the back of our quiet, gently-spoken Doctor Holt, who in turn was leaning over his anesthetized patient. A cacophony of anguish, *of a single voice filled the air with anger, frustration, fury then rage.* If there happened to be a syringe, endotracheal tube, a mouth gag or a simple fountain pen that was recording the patients' progress in our doctor's hand, he would send it flying across the operating room. Aimed at no one in particular but heading rapidly to a bulls-eye.

This tortured, anguished verbal storm would last several minutes, as Doctor Holt's bright shining beet-root red face, and his reddish-pink popping ears finally calmed down back to his pale complexion. During these events his cardio-vascular system must have been under extreme tension as we all thought about how his blood pressure might have been too high to measure, his systolic measurement simply irreversible, and like him beyond recovery and *off the chart.* Should we get him his own trolley to lie on, just in case?

The guilty party, totally responsible for these shouting, vicious outbreaks of slander and atrocious manners, as well as flying objects, it quite clearly appeared innocent, even unaware of the panic, disaster or mental pain that was going on around him, Doctor David Peter Alexander was not yet done.

All the staff in the operating room had on their complete surgical clothing from head to toe and this included the short, above ankle white Wellington Boots.

Those directly assisting in the operation wore the shirt and pants, and long green gowns that covered them from neck to Wellington Boots and tied at the back. However, for those 'circulating' nurses and orderlies, bringing surgical items, counting swabs, resupplying IV bottles or irrigating solutions would stand away from the OR table, being ready to get something and watching progress. The sterile OR gowns worn by the Surgeon and his Assistant, were held up by the circulating nurses as the person essentially wiggled into the gown, and so tied at the back by the circulator. Then, the sterile powdered gloves were pulled over fingers, hands and so on to the cuff of the gown by the operating team. They were as sterile as we could make it.

When our beloved Surgeon and troublemaker entered the operating room through the wrong door and caused these incredible commotions, every staff backed away from the sterile draped patient on the table, back towards the wall. The now calmer Anesthesiologist back on his stool, with the House surgeon facing Doctor Alexander across the table and it was the nurse assisting the surgeon who had to maneuver backwards and towards the foot of the table so that Doctor Alexander could face the house surgeon across the patient whose belly had been opened. The wide retractors gripping the four corners of the surgical site, hence keeping the operating surface clearly visible, a *very open belly,* a chasm of sorts.

Every staff member had been prepared earlier for the vision now before our eyes, but for me this first time was incredulous, breathtaking and even impossible, but here it was. There had been many instances of our Consultants past performances in this same manner, so Sister Marilla Mitchell, the Operating Room Sister, a kindly lady and in full command of her staff and all its equipment, but not however Doctor Alexander. She had given us complete instructions of how to deal with this bizarre Consultants totally inappropriate behavior. It represented a complete loss of sterility, where antiseptic techniques and any pretense of sterility disappeared in a flash.

Sterility disappeared instantly when Doctor Alexander entered through the wrong door. His dress was not the green garb of the operating room, but his well worn suit, that long ago green tweed suit that now showed the wear of the ages, elbows thread bare, worn back collar a darker colour than the surrounding colour and those story telling spots of stains gently mingling into the fading green tweed fabric.

He came into the operating room with his cigarette in full display upon his upper left lip which showed a small circle of red as he inhaled, perhaps unconsciously to get an extra spot of nicotine stimulus into his waiting brain.

It seemed like a *comedy of errors* to me, seeing this for the first time. The surgical opposites of sterility to the maximum versus sepsis waiting to happen!

This cigarette smoking, street clothed surgeon with unwashed hands (but of great repute) now stood next to the fully draped patient on the table. It was as if he was in the morgue, standing over a deceased patient where sterility no longer mattered. He would look into the wide-open surgical cavity and ask his Houseman Surgeon if they were any signs of free hemorrhaging blood, or seeing discoloration from a gangrenous appendix or even a twisted small intestine. Perhaps he would suggest a purse string suture or an anastomosis of a transverse colon, and may even suggest a colostomy. This amazing event remembered forever, indelibly imprinted clearly upon mind through wide, amazed eyes that captured the moment-by-moment sights into my memory as clear as any memory ever remembered in this lovely adventurous life of mine.

Doctor Alexander, his brow folding into convoluted lines of quizzical questioning would plunge his fingers, that a few moments ago were stroking his moustache, into the space between the retractors then deep into the abdominal cavity to pick up a length of intestine as he suggested that, "A resection of the gut at this juncture might be the most advantageous course". *He carefully examined this pinkish white tissue of gut now stretched between both hands*, and then carefully put it back in place. Out came his hands again to stroke his moustache!

He did this extraordinary demonstration whilst he still had his cigarette attached or glued to his upper lip, and I saw (to my own horror) that tiny fragments of cigarette ash, fragment by fragment, floated into this gaping surgical cavern of flesh and intestines! The cigarette flakes of ash occasionally catching the powerful OR light from above our heads made the ash fragments seem like Christmas decorations or snowflakes from heaven under a streetlight.

What was probably the most remarkable event of all was that none of these patients ever had any post-operative complications or post-surgical infections. It had to be that Doctor David Peter Alexander was either incredibly blessed or amazingly eccentric?

Whatever he did and however he did it always had the most positive outcome. Perhaps the disappearing ash was the act of a magician. Certainly, everyone in the Operating Room who wore those white Wellington Boots whilst he wore his dirty old brown lace-up leather boots, somehow or other there must have been a connection. Perhaps all of these bizarre oddities were part of his compendium of remarkable attributes. Everyone, professional or otherwise that knew him, must have wondered about the world he lived in and the balance he kept between his private world and ours.

One special House Surgeon, that appeared to have an uncanny knack of anticipating Doctor Alexander's odd behavior was Doctor Rajeev Singh. Doctor Singh had originally come from the Jamshedpur region of India, who after completing his medical school in New Delhi, came to Edinburgh University and its associated hospitals to complete a surgical fellowship. From there he had finally found his way to our majestic Fortress hospital as a Surgical Resident, and later became our Surgical Houseman.

This Indian Physician had had a wonderfully blessed life. Coming from the central part of the Punjab State, a wealthy family of 3 other older brothers and 2 sisters who were younger than he. His father was a successful banker and his mother a university teacher. During holiday periods, after grueling scholastic demands, the family would spend several weeks at a beachside residence in Goa on India's west coast. It was an expensive but memorable holiday for this large family. Doctor Singh knew his recent British history particularly and the events leading up to Jawaharlal Nehru becoming the first Prime Minister of India in 1947. Although the British had left Indian, Doctor Singh pleaded that they would come back and repair their great railway lines that spread across India which were now falling into disrepair. This was one of the stories that he shared with us whilst he was performing a simple surgery on his own and using one of the Student Nurses as his assistant. Showing his great sense of humour, as he pretended to be a travelling tea salesman stuck on a train waiting for a mechanic to mend a broken train track. Doctor Singh became our *'resident historian and storyteller'*. Whenever there was a surgery that he had to perform, and it was relatively uncomplicated he would with great dexterity do the surgery whilst telling us yet another story of Prime Minister Nehru practicing Law at the Inns of Court, in London, wearing his Barristers wig. An Indian wearing a wig, he could not believe it. He joked that he should have worn that very same wig at his Inauguration as India's Prime Minister.

I enjoyed this opportunity of mimicking his Indian voice since I had already paid a lot of attention to Peter Sellars in both his wonderful films and of course, in the 'The Goon Show'. Almost all the male nurses could imitate his fine Indian voice too, those expressions, the enunciating and copying those verbal Indian spoken characteristics, which became second nature especially after getting used to Doctor Dinesh Malhotra voice as well. So when we called a female nurse or lab technologist, or anyone in a different department and pretended to be Doctor Singh and give some outrageous orders. Finally, after several weeks he became aware of our ruse, so to end our pranks, he would speak Hindi to the person he was calling then switch to English to verify that it really was himself.

He was a good man and probably knew of our misdemeanors with trying to copy his Indian-English accent. He did have a great sense of humor generally, well almost, and he did laugh or smile at our jokes in the quiet times of evening and night shifts when he was on call. Doctor Singh, fondly reminded us that within his family heritage were both warriors and kings and told us not to be surprised he if called upon them to deal with our Peter Sellars-Rajeev Singh imitations.

Looking back on all these remarkable live images it seemed to me, that almost all the Indian physicians had brilliant academic memories, they could write or verbally share with us great depths of any medical or surgical disease, their treatment and related pathology, but, generally it seemed their technical skills were still being acquired, a wonderful group of men.

CHAPTER 4

Specialty Clinics

'Parisienne' Model, Venereal Diseases (the 'Claps' Room)

The Student Nurses kindly called this particular clinic the *Claps Room*. 'Claps' being the general term for Syphilis, Gonorrhea's and every other type of venereal infection that mankind can image. It even included the constant flow of those clingy little creatures, the lice family and their friends.

Our opportunity came in our second year and again in our third year of our Nursing Education to be assigned to this somewhat shadowy and mysterious clinic.

Before actually being assigned to this Clinic there were stories upon stories of patients making up a vast array of females from superbly beautiful women to tragic old and weary women with great odours and sores. With men once full of vigour and muscular vitality to graying, bent and broken bodies in the final stages of this ravenous, destructive contact venereal disease. So it was, the presence of the Claps Clinic and all that entered there.

Coming into the Clinic our patients were dressed in a wide array of clothing from business suits, working overalls to very old and well worn, highly stained shirts, pants and dresses and for all these accidental or otherwise patients, no matter what their clothing was, we secretly wished for an instant magical incinerator, or perhaps even a super powerful, highly concentrated antiseptic spray that would cover their head to toes in a single push of the button! And so, *poof* clean shinning bodies, rather than the sights before us.

Doctor Eric Frost, who was no more Irish than his name might suggest, but was a big, muscle bristling Aussie from Perth. His parents were a Norwegian father and Spanish mother, and he ruled supreme in this *His* Clinic. His voice could be either stern or gruff or remarkable quiet and soothing, it seemed a necessity in this clinic. I was asked several times when new patients arrived how he had arrived at a lovely Irish name rather than a Norse name like 'Olaf Jansen Tordenskold', but that remained a mystery.

The Clinic day began at seven am, earlier than all the other clinics, probably because Doctor Frost did not do Grand Rounds or even Ward Rounds, so if a patient needed hospitalization, he simply referred them to the other consultants. Likewise, if a consultant needed a patient to be seen by Doctor Frost, then they would be transported to the Clinic. His patients would line up, actually filling the thirty or so seats of this waiting room, no privacy, everybody saw everybody else. Patients were here both for their first visit or coming in more frequently for assessment of their disease, which was ravaging body, mind and spirit. Some patients had been coming in for many and years usually those who had ignored their disease in its early stages, hoping it would go away or by a mere miracle the infective, purulent discharge would somehow stop. Those who did ignore those obvious signs and symptoms were the patients now in their later stages of the disease that actually looked haggard and ill. Some were blind or blindness was rapidly approaching, some were frail and needed assistance walking or they stumbled as they slithered there feet, even aided by sturdy walking sticks, or someone's firm shoulder

Every patient was assessed from each of the basic disciplines of medicine. Venereal Diseases required the skills of an Infectious Disease Specialist, an Internal Medicine physician, a Neurologist, an Urologist, a Dermatologist and occasionally the skills of an Ophthalmologist or an Endocrinologist.

Our Claps Doctor was a whiz in all these areas of diagnosis and treatment; it was second nature for him to actually diagnose a new patient before they had spoken their first sentence. He was a very keen observer of the 'human condition', especially as they trembled sitting there in front of him. He never used a desk so his chair faced the patients' chair and it was this close proximity that created extra anxiety in his patients, purposefully done. He wanted the truth, their story, their connections and the facts for his follow-up of who else he needed to contact, stopping *THIS* disease is no easy matter!

The new patients, were almost always, dramatically embarrassed when they came to us. Since they had already been diagnosed of the disease by their own family doctor. That physician then referred them to our VD clinic. It was generally known by our local townsfolk population that if you ever contracted any of these diseases you would end up in the Claps Clinic.

Those first few minutes of an initial visit were somewhat overbearing, embarrassing, causing blushing cheeks to a brilliant bright red, or dry mouths, no eye contact, and stuttering, inaudible voices. From the ladies came cries, tears of anguish and from everyone came guilt, fear and an overwhelming desire to blame some else.

We needed the guilt and blame from all our patients, we needed to find the source, the carriers or carrier spreader of these communicable diseases so we could send out the public health nurses to bring them in for treatment. We needed to be in control of the disease otherwise the disease would be like a rampant lion devouring our community. Guilty people could be family members, neighbors or work pals, possibly someone on your sports team or a college chum. The contact could be a one-time meeting or multiple events, a meeting in another town or even country, a person you might have suspected or not. We would send out the health investigators.

As nurses we had to keep both a serious face for the doctor and his patient as we assisted them both, and we also had to have an almost sustained sense of humor, otherwise the grave circumstances and the abject misery, and indeed, for those in the final days of their lives, that sense of finality- a sadness that seemed so intense, their hope was gone! There were several patients, all of them old timers to our clinic who did have a rare sense of humour, these patients were a welcome break for a warm smile and even occasional laughter from a joke that broke the continuum of sad hearts and faces; they were the ones too, who called our clinic, 'The Claps Clinic of Choice'. In particular there was our blond, blue eyed beauty patient, she was a knockout, a pin-up girl of the highest order, and every single Male Nurse whose duty brought them through the claps clinic, looked at this true blond as a delight to behold, to admire-and we all did, perhaps even to having secret desires to get to know her better, much better. But stop! Here, true beauty was only skin deep, for she was in her fourth year of treatment and had ignored her vaginal discharges for seven months in the beginning before seeking treatment. This meant she was still a possible carrier of this dreaded *lurge*, my nickname for an in-treatment venereal disease. For the sake of her privacy, when we chatted about her, and that was quite a lot both inside and outside of the clinic we called her Simone. The idea was to suggest a name for her, that of a beauty of some mystique, a woman who moved with all the elegance of a Parisienne Model, a woman who simply by looking at you melted all your resolve. Since we knew that her whole presence in the waiting room and examining rooms brought about an admiring bounty of glances and a particularly noticeable quiet, amongst the ladies in the waiting room as they looked, perhaps even admired this beauty within their midst. Then, a moment later realizing where they all were, would whisper critical comments to their companions or neighbors next to them in a jealous retort. The men were attentively amiable, friendly and eyeing every inch of this probable Hollywood Starlet, this Lady of Beauty, indeed, she did move with grace and elegance of those Parisienne Models!

However, within this lovely outward beauty, we knew beyond a shadow of a doubt there was a woman who was hurting physically, emotionally and spiritually from her life changing diagnosis. Looking at her face she never showed her deep distress for she hid it well. For those of us working in the clinic and knowing her History and Physical medical chart, her diagnosis and prognosis, and the scars upon her body and mind we felt a special sadness for her. It's a disease that can show itself quickly or lie dormant for some time. It's a disease that mimics other diseases, a terror to deal with.

Reading her chart, with the laboratory results and the likely prognosis we could feel this tragic sadness for her. Her disease, it seemed had come from a 'one night stand', apparently uncharacteristic for her, she had been away from home on a specialized course in Oceanographic Research in Portsmouth. At this Naval Port she had met a naval officer, who had Syphilis (she learned later). They had said their 'good-byes' in the morning light, and weeks later her vaginal discharge began after lower abdominal pain, itching and general discomfort. Emotionally distraught and trying to deal with her foolishness and the options she may have, time passed!

Apparently it took her several weeks even after seeing the first telltale vaginal sores for her to seek medical advice, the bathing, sponging and using disinfectant pads she had tried, had not worked. She had a Venereal Disease.

She was not alone in this similar story, many a wayward partner gone for an overnight business meeting, and so succumbing to an illicit brief affair, had his or her life changed. Weeks or sometimes months later in a sudden or surprising appearance of sores, or rashes on lips and in or around the sexual organs or a urinary discharge that spells the life changing diagnosis of venereal disease.

Occasionally children would accompany and guide their parent into our clinic. The parent who had had the disease for many years and was now in the chronic stage of Syphilis where blindness, or the debilitating progress had destroyed nervous systems, or joints and bony structures so that walking was now just a series of slow shuffling movements or an unstable hobble at best.

There were, for a brief time, young twin boys both who had both contacted the venereal disease from their mother, a mother either lacking in care or common sense. Perhaps we guessed the reason was to create a massive sense of guilt upon the father, to make him pay for the disaster he had brought upon her. The family seemed quite well off financially and seemed like they had everything, they came from the wealthier side of town. The husband had run his own hardware store business for years but now he was gone, leaving this family in physical and mental turmoil, and needed our help.

Although the Public Health Department went looking for this husband he was never 'found'. We never saw the husband nor did we know if he was the primary contact for his wife's disease. The wife blamed him completely for her disease and therefore the disease she gave to her twin children during her pregnancy, which could have killed the babies in utero. This mother had learned about her husband's venereal disease via a public health worker from a neighboring town, but the husband remained stubborn about any treatment since he neither saw nor felt any signs of the disease. The birth defects for the children affected their eyes and ears, and they had a nervous twitching of their shoulders. The mother for her part, had an ongoing inconsistency with her own treatment and that for her children, she was never clear of the disease symptoms. She remained an active contact, and Doctor Frost our claps doctor was convinced she had infected other male contacts, whether lovers or occasional contacts but she was, or became, a very unwilling and foolish woman, this was a mother as well who had infected her two twin sons during pregnancy, or possibly at childbirth with an infected birth canal to the neonates eyes, her behavior seemed incredibly hostile and destructive. Doctor Frost, social workers and the public health people who were responsible for tracking down VD contacts by trying to first encourage, then if necessary bully them into giving names or places where the disease may have come from, they never had any success with this mother of two, amazing that Doctor Frost's voice of gentle persuasion to a noisy demanding authoritative bark still had no effect, nor did she seem particularly embarrassed by him.

We had a menagerie of characters that would probably keep a comedian in great material for years to come. There was Gerald, a magician who had performed on the South Shore Pier in Blackpool's holiday town. A well-known figure for many years on the stage, that had numerous affairs with the chorus girls who had succumbed to his charm. Gerald was one of the most amorous characters who led the public health nurses on so many cross-country chases going from contact to contact. It was amazing how many innocent or otherwise, young women were diseased by a single man. Alternatively, on the other hand was how many men could have been infected by a flashing eyed beauty with a Venereal Disease. But it seemed end-less at times that this scourge of sexual contact could bring down at civilization if not abated or if not stopped, it could.

On our patient list was the towns *Spiv*. A 'spiv' was the char-acter who dressed the part of an Edwardian trickster, with his slick black hair glued, it seemed, to his scalp. A carefully manicured pen-cil-thin mustache adorned his face, which actually became the cen-tral focus of his face. He also had, but less noticeable unusually thin eyebrows that were either plucked or shaved. He dressed in a black suit that was far too big for him. The sleeves hid his hands except for the tips of his fingers, showing rather too perfect manicured nails, the shoulders of the suit were perfectly square and the suit was always double-breasted. His white shirt was always spotlessly clean, but again the collar was quite loose even though his black tie-which was also barely more than a piece of string in an open cotton weave material; it was tied in a Windsor knot and tied tight. He adorned his head with a thin styled Trilby felt hat that he usually pulled over his eyes, to give the impression of worldliness, mystery or hidden wealth!

Our Spiv patient had a feminine high pitched voice, which added to his many characteristics, but for all of these odd attributes was the lady that came with him for his clinic appointments, and she was quite dazzling. Her adornments were colourful but simple and attractive. She wore a purple or dark blue ribbon-a huge nicely tied bow affair on her hair at the back of her head, but this didn't spoil her hairstyle and the colour of her ribbon always matched the ankle length silk dress that she wore. As a true Lady, she walked with mea-sured careful steps on high heels, in step and harmony just as her companion Spiv walked. Her voice was the quiet gentle, pleasing tones, of a children's storyteller. Both the Spiv and his lady friend spoke with the local Lancastrian dialect, which seemed strange when you looked at them first before listening to their voices. But, come one-come all!

Then there was Patty, an truly chunky lass, almost twice the size of what she should have been, her frame could not fit into one of our normal chairs so she always sat on a wooden bench by the far wall where we had lots of these wooden benches. Those old wooden benches used frequently for two reasons, one was for the ability to sit fairly comfortably if someone was overweight, but the other main reason was to partially provide an area less visible from the other waiting-room patients. There, anyone could hide their constant flow of tears and sobbing, as well as being less noticeable. No matter where she was, *Patty cried from the moment she entered our clinic until she left it*!

She held a small handkerchief in her left hand and used it constantly to wipe or dab away the rolling teas, that hankie should have been totally soaked, even before she sat in front of Doctor Frost for her monthly consultation, but even during their exchange of words, the tears rolled and the eyes got dabbed. It continued to be a mystery why the crying never ceased, it happened every consultation day, and had continued for the four years when she first came into the Clinic's care; Doctor Frost simply assigned secondary diagnosis of Acute and Chronic Anxiety Depressive Syndrome. Sounded right, but she always refused to see the Psychiatrist, since we were there to keep her Gonorrhea free and her antibiotics flowing she felt she did not want anyone else to bother with.

CHAPTER 5

SURGICAL FLOOR

Bare Bums, 'Oh Not My Breast,' and Gaping Holes.

By 6:00 am on any day, the finest most flavourful coffee came from the kitchen of the Surgical Ward. Doctors going on early rounds to other floors stopped here to get their invigorating, most fragrant coffee whose unique salty taste had earned its maker the title, *The Bean Man*, and this man was Niguel Potter. Niguel, now in his late fifties was a simple no-nonsense surgical orderly who had retired after surviving World War Two in the Parachute Regiment. He had been across the world and back, and he could hold an intelligent conversation with anyone. He made the daily coffee with the touch of a master, but it was that delicate balance of the aged coffee beans with the perfect *pinch of salt* that created both its aroma and taste. *Oh, Bean Man where are you now*? I must have drank many gallons of this energy delivering, tasty brew

After the brief, customary patient report, I and the male Student Nurses moved all the beds from one side of the Ward, swept it clean, laid down a thin layer of wood floor polish, then first smoothed the polish into the floor and by the time the other end of Ward was reached it was time to use the final polishing buffer. This routine was repeated for the other side of the Ward until the beds were back in place then the center of the Ward was swept and polished. I shared in the dusting of tables, desks, bookcases or the extra empty beds, or whatever other furniture might have arrived from other Wards in the past twenty-four hours.

As the Male Nurses swept and polished floors the Female Nurses did the rounds of wet and dry dusting of the window sills, ends of beds, bedside tables and the bed screens, those tall metal framed 'privacy' screens with a cloth material stretched in their frame of which there was a set of four frames attached together with double hinges which meant the four frames could be put together or stretched out to provide, at least a modicum of privacy from one bed to another. Each screen had a balanced set of small wheel's that made each individual screen a well-articulated mechanism for privacy.

These screens were the less-than-adequate privacy curtains separating each patient. Each patient hoped that we had enough screens to go around their bed-and it took three lots of screens to create the barest necessity for privacy. The screens were used for anyone either using the bed pan, a major balancing act itself, to a surgical dressing change that required the bed sheets and pajama's to be removed, baring all of a person's nakedness. There were patients who were dying, who couldn't be moved to a quieter more peaceful room, since there was only one room on each floor that could possibly be used for the privacy of a dying patient, and that was the medication and charting room. This room was a big enough room but totally inadequate for a bed and visiting relatives, besides which, it was quite frequent that we had more than one critical or dying patient and each required their own peaceful corner; but the Ward we did have two corners.

It was also a common sight, for anyone, staff member or visitor to walk down the Ward to a patient at the far end of the Ward and so pass one or two patients surrounded somewhat inadequately by our mobile screens and see through the slits in the screen, the patients in the process of using or coming off those stainless steel bedpans, bare bottoms and all this was not an unusual sight. But, bare bums or not, Nursing and Hospital business got done day in and out!

After the sweeping and polishing, after the wet and dry dusting, the beds were made; precision lining up of the top counterpane on each bed, and each bed carefully in line with the next, where the end of the beds themselves were aligned up to a perfect wood floor board.

We were ready for whatever tyrant Sister, Matron or Assistant Matron might want to inspect of our labors. Student Nurses of both sexes worked on both the Male and Female Wards so there was a normal flow of our own nursing maturity in learning and experiencing *opposite sex* anatomy and physiology. Dealing with your private feelings of sexuality most of the time seemed quite normal, but there were times when situations became funny, or sometimes very embarrassing. I do remember days where overt sexuality was readily guarded and because of it sexual maturity developed earlier. Some of our younger patients of both sexes that I knew, even in their early twenties had enormous difficulty with their own sexuality that caused some of the new nurses to refuse to deal with them, but for the majority of the nurses, sexuality was sexuality, just another day!

Some of the days on the Female Surgical Ward, for my own experience were filled with awe and wonder, with fear and anxiety, with apprehension and excitement, I learned so much of the female bod.

Surgical consultant David Peter Alexander our most revered physician, walked the halls of our mighty Fortress, holding daily rounds after his cup of what seemed prized coffee, where he held brief conversations with Niguel Potter, the lowest person on the Wards *who's who* list, but it was the good old army days of their memories that kept the discussions going. They talked quietly of days gone by in army vernacular of places familiar to each of them whist doing their duty for God and the King.

After coffee, the master followed by his lengthy entourage surged into the Ward. In the Female Ward, as in the Male Ward, if a patient was progressing well and there was nothing to report, he hovered briefly giving a word of encouragement.

Otherwise he would discuss the findings of yesterdays operation, new lab studies, or other Consultants reports, then perhaps he would move from the foot of the bed to be by the patients side, hold a probable trembling hand of this young patient who would already be awaiting news from a biopsy–a breast biopsy or an infected wound report. By Doctor Alexander's non-verbal actions of moving around to the side of the bed, then holding a hand, the patient knew the news was not going to be good.

With a thoughtful stroke of his moustache with one hand and with his other hand would try to be as *hopeful* as possible, saying, "The pathology report is positive and it does show significant cancer cells in the areas of your breast where we did our little surgical intrusion into that lump, and which we removed for you. Its the lump you smartly discovered, *so we must completely remove your left breast*, I'm so very sorry to have do this, but we must, and hopefully this will take away all your cancer. This surgery will give you a good chance to survive and have a longer, happier life; now I want you to discuss this with your family and let me know if you agree".

The patients tears flowed, she gasped for air crying, '*Oh, not my breast, please, please no, not my breast no'*. Sadly this scenario played out many times. Beautiful curvaceous breasts, barely noticeable breasts, sometimes both breasts, young and old breasts were removed with abandon. Were these breast removals, these surgical Mastectomies really necessary? Based on laboratory findings of carcinogenic, cellular involvement in surrounding tissues of the surgical biopsies, the mastectomies needed to be done!

Women whose self-image included how lovely their breasts were, sometimes felt betrayed by their own bodies, sometimes they described a sense of resentment to the doctor, and again there was a feeling of being destroyed as a woman to be loved. In the final analysis the breast was removed because the greater fear, a real and known fear, was that if the breast were not removed then their remaining life would ebb away more quickly and perhaps even painfully. So, Mastectomies were a common, all too common procedure.

Occasionally a young lady of our own age would be admitted, this gave the lads, especially the Male Nurses assigned to Nights the opportunity to do more than necessary Nursing Care of this patient, doing extra vital signs, taking a pulse that lasted far longer than necessary, repeating an oral temperature, then telling this hapless lass that we needed to the axilla temperature (under her arm) because the temperature reading needed further verification. Although we tried to get permission to do a *belly to pubic* shave, prior to surgery, since we shaved everyone going to surgery, but there always seemed be female nurses available to do the pre-operative shaving. The Houseman or Resident surgeon would frequently add to his pre-op orders, *shaving to be done in operating room*. Thereby thwarting our chances to be heroes and so the girls' embarrassment and blushes were saved-we might have blushed too! We had previously decided that the abdominal pain the girl was experiencing would be enough for her to be happy that we would shave her and so she would get to surgery that much quicker but that was a vain and lost idea. In actuality, I never did a female preoperative shaving; my Nursing Career was thus lacking!

Probably the saddest event on the three years of my surgical Ward experience was on the male Ward involving a fourteen-year-old lad. His parents had taken him from family doctor to several different specialists, they had been to the main regional hospital in Manchester, had been referred from pillar to post. And yet there was never a clear resolution to this boy's abdominal pain. A Surgeon in an adjoining town had decided his acute pain, that subsided, then became a dull low abdominal ache that migrated to an abdominal position in his upper left area, perhaps behind his spleen which did not need to be explored immediately, but waited and watched for a while. This surgeon determined that all these aches and pains, both acute and chronic were simply *phantom* pains of a Sub-Acute Appendix, and that the boy was acting like a baby.

Although the boy's white blood count was always high-an expectation of any inflammatory condition, he never had the normal 'telltale' signs of a reaction to the palpation and pressure of McBurney's point, actually a point half way from the right iliac crest to the umbilicus, the belly button, no specific pain there was noted. Finally the surgeon did an extended incision over the appendix, removed a normal, healthy Appendix and supposedly did a brief examination of the Bowels, Intestine and Colon and determined he had a normal, to all 'appearances' abdomen and sewed him back up.

The family brought the boy home after a week of recovery. They were not convinced that the root problem was resolved. They were right. Each physician, apart from the last surgeon, that had seen the boy all determined that he was not *acting out* some emotional trauma, and that indeed he was manifesting real pain, the cause was immediately escaping them.

Three weeks after the appendix had been removed, late one night he awoke in excruciating pain, the parents called the doctor-on-call, an ambulance picked the boy up and he finally arrived on our surgical floor, it was in the very early hours of the morning and he was screaming. I was there that night and assisted with his examination, and although it was a noisy time it was very evident to me, and everyone, that this child was having desperate pains. His wild, high-pitched scream awoke everyone. The Surgical Resident tried forcefully to remove the boy's hands that were grasping his abdomen and only with a nurse holding each hand and arm and myself holding his legs was the surgeon able to attempt to examine the boy's now *board-like* abdomen. The board-like nature of the abdomen is a first major sign of a probable Perforated Bowel, which meant immediate surgical intervention.

Parents rapidly agreed, though distressed and tearful. The Consultant and Anesthesiologist and the Operating Room crew were called, and within the hour our fourteen-year-old boy was on his way into surgery. The Surgical Ward patients got back to sleep as the parents were escorted to the empty Prayer Room in the middle of Fortresses' long corridor. Part of the inconsolable sadness for their only child was not forgiving themselves for allowing the last surgeon to do an unnecessary Appendectomy, and this surgeon not being thorough enough to carefully examine all the abdominal organs, and now their son was undergoing another abdominal surgery with all its extra pain and suffering.

The surgery and recovery time was *over seven hours*. At the six hour point of surgery, when the boy's abdomen was being closed and the three red rubber drains were sutured in place, did the Consultant Surgeon, Doctor Alexander come out and make an effort to console the distraught parents.

The boys' abdomen was opened; it showed a huge amount of adhesions, from the Duodenum, at the tip of the stomach to an area covering the Liver, Kidneys and Spleen, essentially all of the upper abdominal cavity thick with fibrous adhesions. The lower Duodenum, the long intestine, had folded back on to itself, twisted and obstructed; this of course prevented the passage of any food contents. The pressure of this unusual folding back upon itself, twisting and obstructing was causing a cessation of blood to the bowel tissue, giving a dark discolouration to the bowel, *the beginning of gangrene and death.*

A small perforation in the upper part of this bowel, next to the stomach had occurred at some point in time, and the bowels' acid liquids, perhaps with a high acidic level causing these adhesions. The shock of free acid in the peritoneal cavity, the scarring of abdominal contents with adhesion formation, all may have put too much pressure on the peritoneum membrane pulling it in various ways to self heal the invasion of bowel contents but also causing the intense, unremitting pain, and the *board-like abdomen* was the key diagnostic sign and symptom.

This was a major event for an adult to endure but a fourteen year old it seemed an enormous ordeal and tragedy.

The prognosis was grave even from the point of opening the belly. The operation of intricate releasing of the adhesions, cutting away dead bowel and anastomosing separate parts of the bowel together again, bringing another lower part of the bowel up through the abdominal surface to form a colostomy and attaching a drainage bag to it, sponging and irrigating all the abdominal organs, intestines and larger bowel. All this enormous stress on a weakened body of a fourteen-year-old boy!

The youth had lost a large amount blood during the surgery, the 'bleeders' difficult to stop, the belly being opened like a cavernous hole, held open by huge metal retractors, claw-like where they gripped the skin and muscle. This gaping hole was being irrigated constantly with saline then suctioned away creating more shock this little body, then there was the respiratory system being anesthetized for just over six hours, even for a healthy adult this major surgery was a physical trial of great proportion.

The boy did not arrive back to our surgical Ward until almost the day dawned and a new group of nurses arrived.

No surgical intensive care facilities then, so when he arrived back we put him in the first bed in the corner coming into the Ward, this gave him a little more room for his parents to be at his side. His body still and completely limp, his ashen pale face seemed blood-less. His breathing, still from the heavy hours of anaesthetized drugged sleep, was barely moving his lungs; a pediatric oxygen mask covered his nose and mouth.

An intravenous drip hung, going into each arm, so that both arms were secured to boards keeping them immobile. Blood was being transfused slowly into one arm whilst the other had normal saline flowing more rapidly to make up his circulating volume and to improve his blood pressure. Two of the three abdominal wound drains ran down the side of the bed to closed sterilized containers; the third shorter drain simply ended in a huge padded dressing over his huge abdominal wound. A catheter drained his bladder of urine so that we could make an estimated guess how his fluid output was related to the intravenous input, and that his kidneys were still functioning.

After I had taken him back to the surgical floor from the oper-ating room and making him look as peaceful as possible, I went get his parents from the Prayer Room. They both looked exhausted and fearful of what was ahead. Walking down the long, still dark-ened corridor back towards the Surgical Floor and their child's bedside, they were sobbing and could not speak nor could I offer them any solace. At the bedside, the Consultant Doctor Alexander reached out to hold first their hands, and then his arms surrounded their limp shoulders. With sadness in his voice he said, "We have done our very best under the grave circumstances which he was in when he arrived here. *He is very critical*, but we will do our very best for him, and you can visit him any time you desire". His par-ents, trying to make some sense of this now greater crisis, clung to Doctor Alexander for a few more moments before letting him go. Our Consultant, turning to leave for home and sleep, and seemingly uncharacteristically said a parting, *God Bless you all*, then left. The parents then completely broke down weeping over their son's bed. Some patients in the Ward aware of this probable miscarriage of medicine upon a mere boy shed their own tears of sorrow and constantly asked about him.

The parents continued to search for an answer of why their son Keith had not been more quickly diagnosed so he would never have got into this terrible state. They asked all the other doctors, surgeons and other consultants who came in to render an opinion of care, they asked all the nursing staff caring for Keith to explain how these events could happen. They did know that at each doctor visit they had made with their sick child, there must have been documentation that may have led to better treatment for him. But now here he was before them in this possible extreme life threatening disaster!

They never got a satisfactory answer to any of their questions. There seemed no specific event that could pin point and would say, *that's how it began.* Over the next three weeks as we gently cared for him, he got to a point where he could smile at a poor joke. When we dressed then redressed his wound as it opened up again and again, it simply would not heal. The surgeon's wanted an infection free wound before they would attempt to cut away the edges of skin and then re-suture this stubborn gaping wound. His open abdominal cavity never healed, but his manner and courage never wavered, he looked into his *body wound* as he called it, at each dressing and simply frowned as he asked the nurse doing the dressing, *"When do you think it will heal?"*

The older male patients on the Ward would, without fail, stop by his bedside and try to be as light hearted as they could, asking about him being on a football team, the position he played, school he went to, what he wanted to be when he grew up and left school? They told him simple jokes and got him to smile. They had their relatives stop by his bedside and chat about family happenings, in all these gentle family discussions Keith tried to smile and be amicable. His parents were there at his bedside during the long hours of the day, they watched as his pale colour became even more sallow and his body weight diminished, his appetite came to an end so we once again increased his IV fluids. They knew that his brave fight for life was slowly and with a certainty coming to an end. Each time they said their *'goodbyes'* at the end of the day they feared it was their last.

In the three weeks we cared for him, it seemed that everybody physically involved with him, had a special warm and loving bond, and even other hospital staff members from all areas of the hospital would visit and ask about him and his parents. All the other surgical floor patients seemed to be aware that his life was ebbing away as they tried their best to be kind and gently respectful of Keith's parents. Remarkably, on the day before he died, his now sunken cheeks showed some blushing pink colour to adorn that pallid white face of his, somehow he seemed more cheerful too as he said his hello's. This for this little fellow called Keith- *this was his peace before the storm.*

He died so quietly in that same corner of the Ward he had been brought to after surgery. His Dad and his Mum were at his side holding his bony, small and cold hands as his hard working heart stopped forever. Tears flowed not just from them but also from our Student Nurses male and female together, and probably from many of the male patients on that Ward that night. It was a sad and gloomy night that would be remembered.

Long after Keith was gone, we talked about this special brave little boy and his sadly grieving and distraught parents who constantly thanked us for the loving care we gave him. I wondered too, if our modern medicine really had helped or hindered him, since none of the surgeries and none of the antibiotic drugs ever seemed to work for him.

On a different lighter subject, I had a Student Male Nurse accomplice who delighted in creating a more adventurous realm to our hospital Fortress's night shift. We wanted to keep our senior members of the hospital's administration on their toes, or even on their knees... to give them a real, or even supposed dilemma to deal with when they arrived on Monday morning's to begin a brand new week, with more than the *same old routine* stuff.

We had discovered a way to breach the kitchens well locked substantial doors, and once into the kitchen we had access to the dining room where dignity, seniority and rigorous orderliness ruled this Hall of Gastronomic excitement. In the still dark hours before dawn the driver and his assistant would deliver fresh food items. They had a key to open the kitchens sturdy door, they then blocked it open the door knowing that if the door closed it automatically locked, so once they were well inside the kitchen, we would tape over the protruding bolt pulling it back into its housing, then plugged the bolts' fairly deep hole on the door frame with lots of black ink soaked cotton wool-so that unless you looked very carefully the black hole still looked black. The men didn't seem to notice that the lock didn't 'click' as the heavy door closed after them.

This lovely prank worked twice. Once inside we first we rearranged all the tables so that the head table was now at the opposite end of the dining hall and soon we moved all of the chairs out and hid them in an overflow Orthopedic Ward. We took all the silverware, tablecloths and napkins, placing them into a large Post Box, not far from the Assistant Matrons Office. The postman wouldn't open the box till 11:00 am; so this was a single stroke of genius, no breakfast utensils. Nobody would be able to determine when the prank happened-either on a Friday, Saturday or Sunday or on evenings, nights or early mornings so finger pointing would be more difficult. And we were never suspected!

Our second major foray into the kitchen, some couple of months later, using the same lock blocking technique, was to remove all the pots, pans, ladles, knives and kettles, everything that seemed to be used for preparing food. This time we ventured further afield to hide our loot and bounty. We hid it across a backyard area, across a small grassy lawn to the gardeners' greenhouse, and since it was never locked it seemed a perfect repository! The little venture did create huge consternation; the cooks and their staff blamed the hapless delivery driver. It seemed everyone in every administrative position was summoned to the hospital, oh joy and we were never discovered again, lucky for us.

However, we were discovered on one of our more visible antics. In the darkness of the night, on the very dimly lit and now at night, the noisy tiled floor corridor- especially if someone was wearing leather shoes, the noise of the footsteps could be heard down the whole length of the corridor. The echoes down the corridor always seemed eerie especially if only one or two people were walking down it, and in the shadows of this darkened corridor there always appeared to be a mystery of sorts. This main corridor *was* long, appearing as it stretched from our Surgical Ward all the way down to the Operating Room, it even appeared to disappear into its own dark cavern. The surgeons loved to call the Operating Room the *Theatre* so perhaps they were always expecting a great Shakespearian Comedy or an Orchestral Concert performing Mozart, Rachmaninoff or an Opera as they entered. The corridor had many adjoining corridors connected to it, besides hallways, waiting rooms, the Prayer Room and various offices and stairways up or down leading to Nursing Administrators, as Matron or the Hospital Administrator himself. But this was nighttime, and we choose the peace and solitude of the two o'clock hour. *No living person* should be out or about at this time. No operations were being performed, no one was particularly critical and the Supervising Assistant Matron had done her rounds and we were free for two more hours!

Using those lovely huge black capes the female nurses wore when going into the outside colder environment, we surreptitiously borrowed two capes and carefully rounding the hoods over our heads fastening the hood with safety pins, then allowing the wings of the cape to cling close to our bodies, which, using a bandage tightened as a belt, and allowing the bandage ends to hang down, we now in the half light had the silhouette appearance of a Friar, a Monks or even a Priest.

Heads bowed and clasping hands together as if praying we began a slow meditative walk from the Surgical Floor towards the Operating Room. As we very slowly walked we began what might have been a grand Gregorian musical chant, or at least a good effort, much as a priest may use during a more formal service. We sang our own individual chant trying to imitate the most beautiful Latin *or something similar*, our voices, at least to us, were harmonic, Angels may have gently approved. We chanted and our voices echoed down this darkened sanctuary corridor, our own voices and the words creatively proffered forth, seemed to encourage us, to give us the emotional energy to keep chanting and progressing down the corridor. Cloaked with hood, bowed head and folded hands our image from one end of this now reverent corridor to the other end could have been part of a mystery film from the bowels of some ancient castle, or from a Medieval Cathedral offering shelter from the stormy, black night. I thought this chanting harmony of ours was melodious not eerie or chilling, though not expectant of praise from unseen people, for this story was still unfolding.

We have done this two o'clock marching chant several times, and each time successfully completing the distance in both directions to be welcomed back by the Surgical Ward night shift nurses, all two of them. But, as might have been reported by some person lacking any sense of humour, this night we had a waiting surprise. Just over half way down the corridor a short narrow set of stairs led up to the usually uninhabited Prayer Room. As we drew level to this gently hidden area in the darkness of the passageway, out popped the local priest in all of his official religious garb, gesticulating and in a fine Irish voice raised well above our melodious chanting, demanding an instant cessation! *Never to do this again, and you two will be properly disciplined*, he yelled at us. He was really upset, his face glowed red in anger.

We thought he might have planned to stay awake so that he might catch us, especially if a nurse who thought we were being very sacrilegious had informed him. Perhaps after being told of our exploits previously he was anxious to catch and stop us. This Priest had no humour in him, so it was not a surprise when we learned he had formally complained about us to the Matron. Later the Matron set a time for our disciplinary counseling with this humourless Priest.

Dutifully we arrived with perfect punctuality at Matron's office door, we knocked and entered, our Priest of the night was already inside the office and bristling with expectation that we would be thoroughly brought to our unceremonious knees. I believe he became saddened when the matron, after hearing his story then asked him kindly to leave the office, as she wanted to speak and counsel us privately. He left the office dismayed, downtrodden; he would not be there to see us verbally whipped!

The Matron, always a fair nursing administrator, spread her hands fingertip to fingertip, slowly looked up from her desk and surprisingly asked us, "What shall I do with you? You haven't really done anything worthy of, she smiled- a flogging, have you?" *"Perhaps it was your bad harmony?"* She asked again, her voice being normal and quiet, where we had expected her voice to be full of distressed indignation. We understood the message, and replied quietly that it had all been done in gentle fun, and in no way to imitate the priest, which was his criticism of us. So we were forgiven and allowed to go on for another day-or night, but with no more Gregorian Chants at the Two o'clock hour.

The Sister for this Surgical Ward was actually a wonderful old Battle Axe. She was a refined buxom lady with a grand memorable voice, perhaps an opera star or a Lady Warrior Queen of some Persian army in the Ancient of Days. Her name was Sister Lisa Simon, which sounded like a very modern name; I was expecting a name like Henrietta Snodgrass when I first met her, which may sound earlier Victorian, but there she was, as large as life itself!

The first time she yelled my name, pronouncing it perfectly I jumped to a rigid attention. I had arrived on the Ward barely five minutes earlier to introduce my self and for a brief orientation prior to my first full day the following morning. She yelled, I replied by running to her office-an office I would eventually get to know well. *Greenhalgh go and deliver the Stout to everyone*, she proclaimed. I had no idea what she was talking about!

Catching up with me, and pulling on my arm was that older, wiser Staff Nurse Sam Moore. He introduced himself as 'just an old nurse who has been around along time', but he actually struck me as a wise and patient fellow. I came to trust him a lot, he was a great teacher and I remember his first lesson that day, look carefully at everything, before you speak. Fortunately for me, he was my mentor on that Ward, he could diagnose a good 75% of all the patients coming into the Surgical Ward, even whilst they were being rolled into the Ward on the Ambulance's stretcher, and well before the Surgical Houseman showed up. This required many years of careful observation and following through with lab and X-ray studies, but generally he was right.

The *Stout* Sister Simon was yelling to me to go and give, were the bottles of *Guinness Stout* that was given to every adult patient that wanted one. This had been a practice for several years after it was discovered the food value of this nutrient rich Irish beer. The beer was free and it was delivered in the evening, no need to catch the bus and go to your local pub.

Where Sister Simon was the titular head and very obviously the leader of the Surgical Ward and 'all nurses that entered into it'; hers was the voice that mattered. Sam was the calm professional who guided most of the nurses through their Surgical Ward experience and he did it with warmth and kindness, though he did have a sarcastic humour about him. Like Doctor Alexander, Sam was a career smoker. His unique cigarette specialty was that he did not need to touch the cigarette once it was on or between his lips, the cigarette would burn down to its last fraction of an inch then simply extinguish itself! I could never remember him spitting out the tiniest vestiges of tobacco or paper-it disappeared, but where?

Through Sam's instructions on Surgical Ward on each of my three years there, I became adept at listening to Bowel Sounds through the stethoscope, I learned to place either one hand or both hands on a peaceful or painful abdomen, I learned the skill of placing a patient in the perfect position so a spinal tap could be done first time, I could recognize skin or mucous membrane colour's and their changes and by touching a patient's brow with my extended fingers could instinctively know the progression of Haemorhagic shock. These skills of *touch* and *hearing* were combined with the recognition of a variety of smells-most of them unpleasant coming from a patient and then observations from *looking* at conditions of colour and muscle activity, and so a deliberate Nursing Conclusion, a Nursing Diagnosis could be reached. A skill, more an observation I learned, was touching the patients nose with the back of my hand-and *feeling* its still warm or very cold tip, indicating that the patients life was ebbing away rapidly. These were the skills learned at this Fortress Hospital, and the Nurses completing their three-year training there could go out into the world and be Great Nurses. And we were!

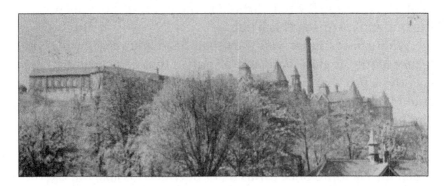

Queens Park Hospital (The 'Fortress'-from Queens Park Lake).

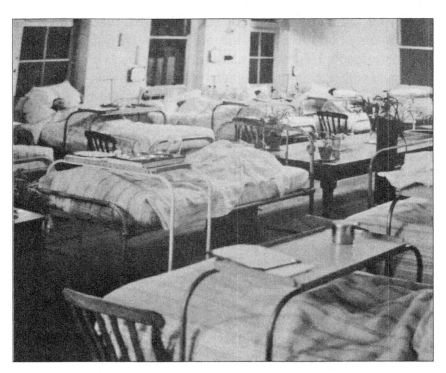

Surgical Ward at night, shows 1 of 3 beds in middle of Ward.

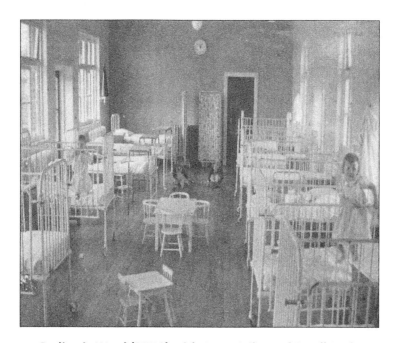

Pediatric Ward (PEDS) with Cots, Cribs and Small Beds.

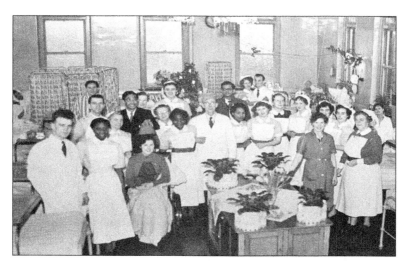

Surgical Ward at Christmas-Surgical and OR staff.

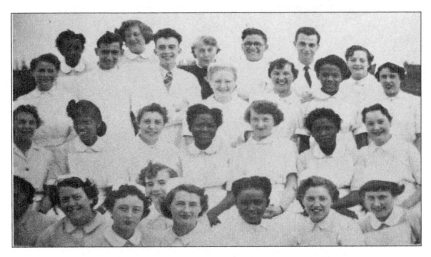

**Park Lee Hospital for 'Invalid Cookery' -group of
Student Nurses with Sister & Staff Nurse.**

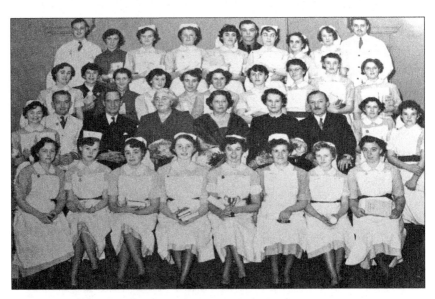

**Graduating Class of Student Nurses to S.R.N. with Matron,
Nursing Tutor & Administrators.**

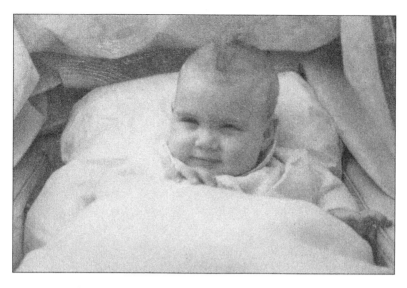

'Baby Anne' in the story, not her real name.

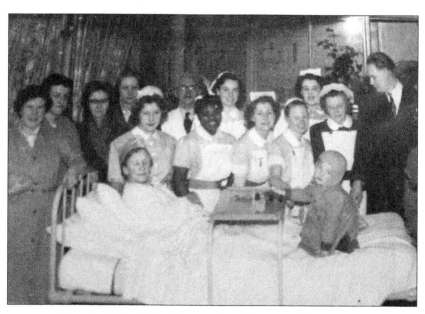

**Surgical Ward Nursing and Auxiliary Staff, Sister 'B',
Staff Nurse 'D', & Resident Surgeon.**

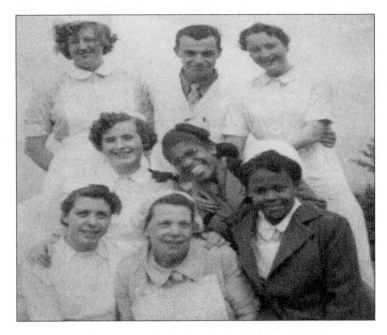

'Invalid Cookery' Class, small group with Author.

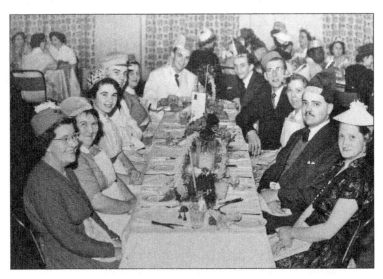

**Hospital Christmas Dinner, Author at head of table,
& some great characters**

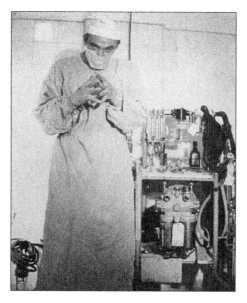

Author-3 years after graduating, in RAF, 'in-charge' of OR at APL Khormaksar Hospital, Aden, Arabia.

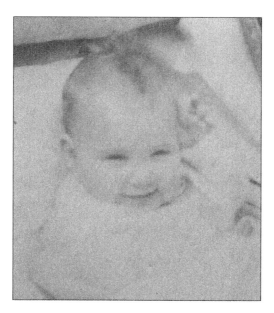

'Baby Anne' happy in her short life.

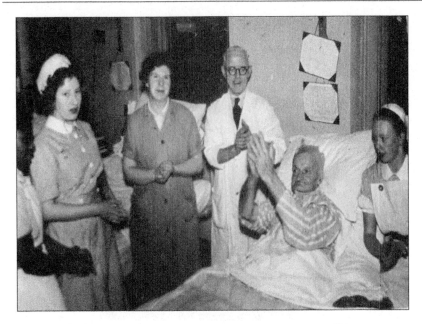

Surgical Ward patient singing & leading nursing staff in a song.

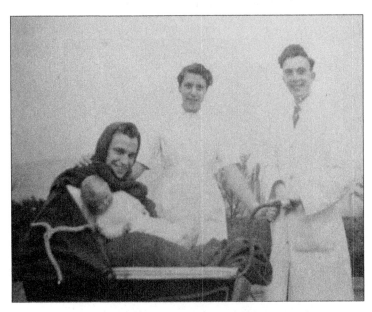

Author in a Pram with a doll & 'Mum and Dad',
rehearsing for a 'skit'.

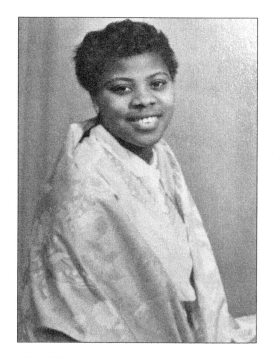

Our Nigerian Princess -Student Nurse.

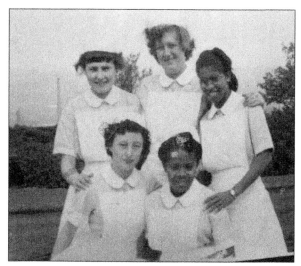

**Student Nurses of Medical Ward, of England,
Ireland & West Indies.**

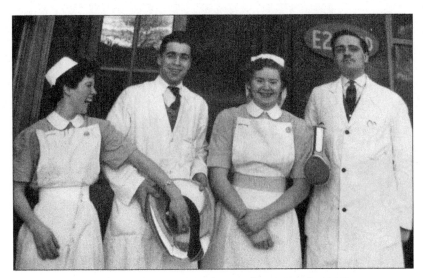

**Joyful Irish Staff Nurse and compliant Student Nurses
with 'instruments'.**

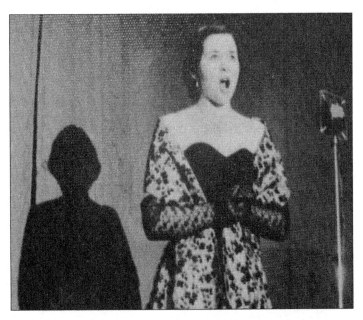

Our Favourite Irish-Student Nurse-songstress 'P'.

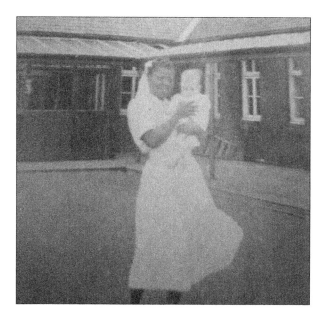

Nigerian Student Nurse holding 'Baby Anne'.

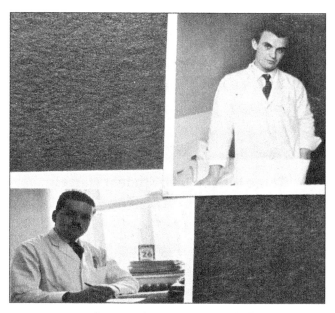

**Author, senior year, upper left;
colleague 'B' in senior year.**

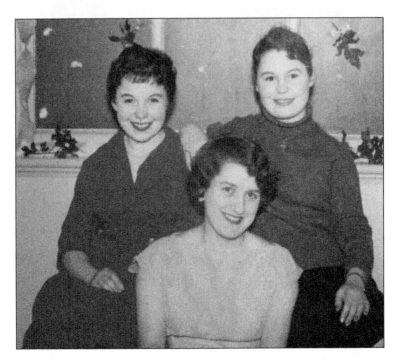

Three Irish Colleen Student Nurses.

CHAPTER 6

CASUALTY

None Dare call it 'a Casualty'

T was' the Realm of Doctor Strangelove and Hob Nail Boots.
Long before the elegant days of ICU, CCU, NICU's or Intensive Care *anything's* it was just simple Pediatrics, Medical, Surgical, Ortho, Casualty, OB, GYN, OR, Clinics and the 'Mental Ward', no kinder reference or titles like 'Psychiatry'. Besides these Specialties, and on the grounds of this Fortress Hospital, we had a large Geriatric Hospital, which was close to the fairly busy Clinic Building area where on different days of the week, it would be taken over by the specialties of Medicine, Surgery, Obstetrics and so on. This would bring together the Consultant and his staff for their Clinics

If a diagnosis was unclear or perplexing in any of the normal clinics then a more specific investigation was needed, the consultant would refer to the Regional Hospital Center in the larger city of Manchester where the Endocrinologist or Infectious Disease specialists or other key doctors practiced. Sharing the same complex, as the Clinic's was the Casualty Department Each was adjoined with yet another lengthy tiled corridor. It had a large waiting room with old oak benches hard as a rock for everyone to sit on, and since the examining rooms almost surrounded the waiting room, everyone in pain who wanted to make a noise, or cry, or yell, did so with abandon. Like the Clinic, there were times when the sounds coming from the waiting room had the gentle sounds of a piano concerto. Most of the time, however it was the clattering noise of an orchestral hall with out a conductor and its cacophony of loud protesting voices and high pitched shrieks of crying wondering why they had to wait so long and sit on hard miserable benches.

You had to be bleeding, actually bleeding or be cyanotic and purple, and on your last breath of life to get priority treatment.

This was a great place to work on many skills at the same time, and your ability to *stop that wailing noise so you can tell me exactly where it hurts* skills! Occasionally we would borrow one of the Nursing Orderlies from the orthopedic Ward to come over and demand quiet. This was Joshua, 'Josh' and he was proudly from Barbados, his skin was a shiny black ebony, his rippling muscles showed prominently under his green tight orderly uniform smock and his 197 lbs. small but well filled framed of about five foot six was attention getting! When he came over to help he usually stayed and helped for two or three hours in those times of need.

Joshua had served in the Royal Army Medical Corp for 21 years in the Medical Branch ending his career as a sergeant, and when he demanded 'quiet' from this seemingly unruly waiting room—he got it—quickly. Perhaps it was his lovely black face that was adorned by a shock of pure white hair! But everyone listened and even the children were hushed. Peace had come again and we could hear ourselves.

This too, was the world of *Casualty* our emergency department had a unique and ever changing character of its own. It essentially joined the clinic building and had access to the outside world through huge double doors with round windows on each door and beyond that was the covered portico with its semi circular drive way for ambulances to unload their patients. The Consultants, Housemen or Residents appeared on time when we needed them but heading Casualty in every sense of the word was Doctor William Trevor Adcroft, an ex military man of the RAMC (Royal Army Medical Corp).

In many ways he had similar character traits to our Surgical Consultant, Doctor David Peter Alexander where he made everything an adventure and exciting to work with him. There was nothing ordinary that ever happened within these walls whilst I was there; here I found my ultimate element as a Student Nurse. I would gladly do this all over again and again!

Doctor Adcroft had also come a family of physicians who owned a fairly large farming estate in Devon maintaining substantial dairy cattle. So it should not have been a surprise to anyone to see this Casualty physician wearing brown boots, well-worn brown boots, well-worn Army brown boots! They also probably reminded him of his adventurous army career. He loved his profession and had that 'gift' of giving each patient the benefit of simple laboratory tests that he ran on the spot whilst they waited. He was another great example of those Critical Observation Skills by using his natural senses of touch, sight, smell and hearing. Certainly he used his beaten up old stethoscope and his aging red-rubber Reflex Hammer, both of which he kept stuffed into the back pocket of his trousers. Prior to coming to our hospital he had been in the R.A.M.C. (Royal Army Medical Corp) for 15 years, which he had joined immediately after completing medical school.

He apparently had loved Army life, had been stationed in Singapore, Burma, Cyprus and somewhere in East Africa, so had brought with him a colourful past and stories of wild tropical diseases and doing small surgeries in jungles. Why he had left the army, no one knew but perhaps his eccentric ways had been the reason, but our Fortress Hospital had the propensity to be militaristic, so perhaps he would not miss his Army days too much.

Night shift in casualty was an absolute joy for the Male Student Nurses, (the Female Nurses worked only during the day shift). The Male Nurses essentially worked alone through the night, if we needed help it was always close by. On nights we became *nursing physicians extraordinaire*, a title we gave ourselves. On my first night with Doctor Adcroft, it was a night never to be forgotten, he counted on all of us to be his eyes, and ears, hands and I believe his diagnostic and therapeutic extensions of himself. We were his and he belonged to us, how could you have anything better than this. Once again, this was Nurses Training of the most exotic.

To reach Casualty from his office and sleeping room, Doctor Adcroft had to walk down yet another green tiled corridor of about forty yards. At night, this was significant since on his brown boots he had the metal heel and toe pieces on these well-worn boots. One of the horse-shoe shaped metal sole supports had worn loose, which meant that when he walked the metal piece 'clipped' like an extra echo to this steps. We could hear him clipping' down the corridor from the moment he left his room. But this was just the beginning of this rare mans appearance, dress and character.

Long before it was vogue to wear an OR shirt, that green short sleeved, v-shaped neckline shirt, this was his twenty-four hour a day garb. Occasionally he switched from his khaki army pants to heavy black canvas trousers. He was a hairy man and this was instantly obvious when anyone stood before him, since tumbling out of his shirt was his black curly chest hair, and there was enough of it to share around. This black haired man was very hairy!

Doctor Adcroft usually didn't shave from week to week, so by the end of a week he had the fine beginnings of a black stubbly moustache and beard. To meet him for a first time, if you were not aware of him, it was quite a shock! It became a shock for many timid, often frightened mothers bringing into Casualty their child already whimpering in pain. Then, to be instantly confronted by this odd looking character who was now their Doctor wearing what may have been perceived a pajama top! This was surprise number one. Frequently his voice was not the most gentle, especially if we had awaked him in the early morning hours after he had just gone to bed from the last patient. We did try and warn the family about Doctor Adcroft's appearance before he arrived in front of them. His black curly hair did get trimmed at the back, but in front, curls cascaded over his forehead and it was obvious from day to day, that this dense forest of hair never saw a brush or comb. And so it was, at night in the gloom of electric lights he presented an image of a fearful ogre, this was surprise number two. He was not the kindly, patient and understanding type of a practiced family physician, which the hurting patients coming into Casualty would have certainly preferred.

In spite of his darkly old and gruff appearance, he was a gifted diagnostician. His senses and his human observations of listening carefully to a verbal complaint, or to recognize heart sounds, or listening to chest with a struggling pair of lungs, and feeling with the touch of his fingers upon cold moist skin, or the hand depressing a certain area of the abdomen, and getting specific reactions. His ability to recognize all the differing odor or smells of a human body, as breath and skin odours, or understanding the nature of infected sores and wounds. When he looked at his patient he saw beyond the obvious, he noticed a myriad of skin colour changes, muscles tensing, guarding or so tight that below them a major catastrophic event was becoming life threatening.

Whether he ever used his tasting skills I never knew-nor cared to! The lads of our Nursing band of brothers, after hearing great stories and having those incredible unique 'do it yourself experiences' under Doctor Adcroft's authority, everyone looked forward with great anticipation to working with him.

My rotation to Casualty arrived; I had joy in my heart and great expectation in my spirit. That first night in Casualty was busy when I arrived at 10:00pm but it soon cleared as patients were treated, bandaged, medicated or referred to specialists on another later day.

When all the patients were gone Doctor Adcroft had his interview with me. Mainly, he was interested in why I was here, why was I a nurse, what made me decide to come to Casualty (apart from the obvious answers of it's my turn to rotate here). He was, I think impressed by my story of being in the Boy Scouts and being on the St. John's Ambulance Brigade Team and being a leader of our team in those competitions. These competitions were actually a brilliant pre-cursor to Nursing, for at our young age 14 or 15 years old to be involved with medical emergencies, and how to deal with them. My own particular story was, where our team won the regional competitions. We were a three man team, and so coming upon a man and woman both lying in the set-up street, the woman lying twisted and the man bleeding from a huge abdominal open wound and with a piece of glass protruding from his bleeding neck. The make up team doing very realistic jobs of these vehicular and related accidents.

As a team leader it was my job to *treat* these patients as if no one else would be available for some time. We were the First Aid Team and first to arrive. We needed to act quickly, the jagged piece of glass protruding from the left side of his neck bleeding profusely, as well as the belly wound a large cut showing skin and muscles opened to the air, but bleeding less than the neck wound so this could be dealt with secondarily.

In approaching the accident I yelled to a passer by to call an ambulance or a doctor or both, if they could get one. I determined the man had a decent strength but rapid pulse; he had slow shallow respirations, however he was alive but was bleeding profusely. The glass coming out of the wound would be the problem. I knew that glass had to stay there! So I quickly created a circular bulky bandage from the Boy Scout necktie around my neck and placed it very carefully over the glass and onto the wound putting pressure on the wound but away from the glass. After completing this, then covering the abdominal wound, I declared I had stopped the free flow of blood and both his pulse and respirations were normalizing. It was a competition so we saved the patient and won the day.

This true story of mine seemed to make Doctor Adcroft believe I was ready for the *Greater good of Casualty* their solutions and experiments. The aspects of experiments gave me a profoundly uneasy feeling-until I knew what he meant.

Doctor Adcroft's plan for me was pretty much the same plan he used for the previous Male Nurses coming into Casualty, and under his graphic directions, his aspirations, and his desire to get some midnight sleep.

He taught me how to suture any minor wound. He taught me how to take a simple x-ray, develop it then read the result of the film. Reading the film was simply based on a rather beautifully illustrated large poster of our human skeleton, and surrounding the skeleton in smaller illustrations how each bone was interconnected with its companion bone and it showed how a minor fracture appeared on the x-ray, as well as how a minor dislocation would look. This seemed remarkably academic and medically futuristic even for a third year Student Nurse, but hey this is the adventure we *signed up* for, so to speak. If Doctor Adcroft trusted our innate ability to do comparative analysis between the x-ray just developed and this lovely well-detailed anatomy and basic fractures poster, then we could do it. If there would be a questionable treatment we made during the night when he was sleeping, and the patient had gone home, no problem, we could call them back, and if they did not have a telephone we would call the police department, and they would bring them in.

For the problems of a dislocation of an arm or a leg Doctor Adcroft gave us a 15 minute course on how to apply a Plaster-of-Paris cast around the limb to immobilize it after repositioning it to normalcy. What? Well we could do that too. So for our first patient to come into Casualty with either or both a wound needing suturing or an obvious arm or leg that was dislocated, he would be there to instruct an encourage us, showing us carefully how to make the repairs to the dislocated part, and when they did arrive, we watched, then Plaster-of-Paris' them. Doctor Adcroft, in his wisdom or foresight told us not to suture or x-ray any major head trauma until he had first done a thorough exam and investigation of how the trauma occurred. If it was some other body part and a simple laceration, we were free to suture up a storm, and we did. There was always a great supply of suture needles, straight or curved with sutures of silk or various catgut sutures.

After my first night of instructions from Doctor Adcroft I was on my own. I sutured and sutured, I became an expert tailor of human flesh. I also became a master of the Plaster-of-Paris cast room. With the x-rays I had taken now put up into the viewing box on the cast room wall, I must have looked like a *pro* well, I felt like it anyway, and no one was looking either.

A bonus to this suturing and plastering was that when we had a lovely young lady, even with her parents, who presented into Casualty with the requisite arm or leg injury that required our artistic skills it always took a little longer since we had naked skin before our eyes that needed extra attention from our eyes, so did the handling a lovely limb need gentle nursing care! And generally these lovely lasses looked upon us as healing knights as they lay upon our examining table in Casualty, or on upon Plaster-of-Paris table in the Cast Room. It was amazing just how much time it took on these occasions, and by then, we had given the parents a cup of tea, sat them down in the waiting room, and with no other patients waiting to be seen, the night was ours-*for care*, of course.

There was really only one occasion, when our resident maestro Casualty Physician actually struck terror into the hearts of some poor family people coming into our casualty department at the unkind hour of two-thirty in the early morning. During this wet and dreary night, even from the inside we could hear the thunder claps outside as the latest heavy rainfall banged on our single story roof. This late November it was cold with a biting sharp wind to add to the misery of the rain. If you didn't own a car, then there was no choice but to rely on a kind neighbor or the call for a taxi service. No buses or other local service ran through the night hours, otherwise you were walking.

This couple, rain soaked and bedraggled, rather old to be parents in their late forties brought in their only child a little girl who was small for her three years, she had a constant irritating wheezy cough, had a feverish pyrexial temperature of one hundred and two as well as being very lethargic and even appeared to be under nourished. Indeed she even looked pale and quite sick to an untrained eye. Both parents were frantic with their barrage of questions, and were genuinely concerned and worried about her condition. Their voices sometimes loud sometimes a whisper, questioning if what they had been doing for her was right, or was it making her worse. As the little girl began shivering violently after I had removed her clothes to take her vital signs and listen to her breathing sounds, I became quite anxious myself for her, and with the parents on each side of the stretcher, now with extra blankets from our warmer-cabinet covering the girl, I quickly moved down the corridor to Doctor Adcroft sleeping room, and knocking perhaps a little more aggressively than necessary, I heard the growl of a reply from within.

I shouted more than spoke that I needed him *now*.

Foolishly in my haste, I had forgot to warn them about our doctor's appearance, but it was too late, perhaps because of my more than usual urgency Doctor Adcroft came quickly. He was obviously annoyed at me for waking him up after only thirty minutes of sleep from the last patient.

His black appearance coupled with the noise of his 'metal on tile' noise of his boots, hurriedly pulled onto his feet were still untied, these loosely fitting boots making an even noisier approach than usual was the introduction this fragile family had of what must have been an *apparition of some black haired angry being* from the darken corridors of this Fortress!

Doctor Adcroft didn't quietly enquire what the problem was, he bellowed making both his curly black hair do a fandango on his forehead and the unsightly bushy chest hair seemingly move in rhythm as they squired over his open shirt. His questioning bellow of *"what are you doing to this child"* brought the two parents into cries of anguish, feeling guilty of some misdeed. They both cried quietly as tears flooded down their cheeks, and the child, now hearing both her father and mother crying increased her own volume of noise.

It was a rare cacophony of the night that I had not heard before in Casualty. A foursome of raised voices, Parents, Child and Doctor, it had to stop. Calm had to come from somewhere, so I picked up the child and held her protectively, only then did other three adults calm down back to a realization of why we were there, for this little girl, and she needed all three of them.

Putting the child back down on the exam table I handed Doctor Adcroft his stethoscope, and moved away to where I now stood behind the parents and asked them to step back a little, Quietly I tried to explain to them the doctors appearance and his unusual bad bedside manner, having had no real sleep for fourteen hours and then, my waking him up after he had just gone back to bed and began sleeping.

They were quieter now and I thought quite reasonable under these circumstances, they gave him the benefit of the doubt after thoroughly examining the child, and made his diagnosis of 'Sever Pneumonia in both Lungs', where upon he picked up the child holding her on his shoulder rocking her gently and covering her with one of the blankets. With this three-year-old little girl cradled on his shoulder Doctor Adcroft carried the child to the Pediatric Ward that was some good distance from the Casualty department. With the clipping sound of his army boots and its one loose metal horseshoe stud hitting the cold tile of the corridor floor it was the only sound to be heard. The parents now more at peace followed behind him. Two hours later, after their daughter had been given antibiotics and fluids, then finally had fallen into an exhausted sleep did they walk back into the Casualty Department to thank me and hug me for being a *real nurse*. What a lovely way to say 'we appreciate you and thank you'.

That morning as I left for home, I felt a real hero. I felt that all my Nurses training had prepared me for such eventualities. Now I fully understood why so many of our staff members had given the ominous title of Doctor Strangelove to Doctor William Trevor Adcroft. This distinguished fascinating title of Doctor Strangelove, had itself the epitome eccentricity, of changing characteristics, of both the highs and lows of the human condition, but we steered away from the less dramatic idea of schizophrenia. But perhaps, because we gained so much experience from him we let the better idea of *bizarrely eccentric* be his *'modus operandi'*.

Interestingly, a World War Two, a Royal Air Force Flight Lieutenant who had been a Navigator in Bomber Command, called Peter George had written a book called 'Pattern of Death' in 1954, and after writing that, became fascinated with the specter of Nuclear armaments. By 1958 he had written a book called *'Red Alert'*, it was this story that became the *Doctor Strangelove* in the film of the same name. The story of a very wild and madly eccentric character, but we had given our eccentric Doctor the title first!

Casualty Department through the dark nights, brought in a constant flow of cuts and skin tears that I carefully and meticulously sutured. Bone dislocations of fingers, hands, elbows, knees, ankles, or feet I carefully cradled and then laid on the table for the x-rays, then developing them, reading them-to my best ability. I again cradled these hands, arms or legs bones and wrapped them in the white Plaster-of-Paris bandages that became the solid casts. My brilliant technique, and artistic sculptural jobs I would always think to myself what a *great technician of the trade* I am, you were meant for this! Or was this just my pride?

Long after my Casualty Nursing experience was over, which had been so powerful, I wondered time and again, with an inner smile that only I knew, if there were any of my old ex-patients walking around with a 'not-quite' so perfect suture line where each side of the wound should line up with the other, or where a finger or limb was slightly bent out of alignment due to my 'innocent' misreading of the x-ray or placing the limb in the not-so perfect position as I applied the Plaster-of-Paris cast! (But great for a Boy Scout who was always *Prepared*...and preparing for greater things.)

Oh, these days never to be repeated with the same joy and excitement, *Casualty where are you now*? And to those lovely old and young people wandering around the town and countryside who may have a slightly uneven scar on their body, or a limb, finger, or toe that was set at an odd angle, and never came back to its normal shape! *I'm sorry*, but you did get loving, caring treatment whilst I tended to your discomfort, so hopefully that all balances out, and you are still alive to tell the story.

To the outside world and ruling over all the varietal departments of Casualty and the Clinics, where at the evening hours and into darkness was the bright shining *emblem of hope* light that shone its simple message, the big foot high red letters on a gleaming white background read *CASUALTY* to the world outside. The ruler of this domain was the petite twenty-seven years old Sister Linda Forester. Sister Forester had been in charge of casualty for two years before my arrival in her department, but as far as all the Male Nurses that came to work on the Night Shift were concerned, she was the most well known of all the Sisters, in no small part because she was definitely the most attractive. She was the most likely female to be chosen by the Nursing journal, *'The Nursing Mirror'*, for both her superb management of this 24-hour a day Casualty department and her sublime beauty. Besides which we all expected that either the *'British Medical Journal'* or *'The Lancet'* to do a significant story on Sister Forester and the efficiency with which the Casualty Department satisfied and resolved all patients with true 'emergent' needs. Our hopes of finding Sister Linda Forester commissioned into the hallowed halls of Nursing; *or to be the next cover girl of that wildly popular magazine*, Tit-Bits, but we are all still waiting. Time may have beaten us to those publications.

Even in my first week at the hospital, as a Cadet Nurse I knew who she was, which department she worked in what time she always chose to be in the Dining Room for lunch, at what time she generally ended her work day, and who her suitors might be. This was part of the underground secret network between all the Male Nurses.

When the conversations of the lads turned to the aspects of beautiful women, her name was always there. We talked of desire, of passion, of a longing to be slightly older so we could have a chance, on an age to age similarity, rather than we being seven and eight years her junior. Secretly, we also longed to be wealthier, where we could ask her out to our yacht for a Mediterranean cruise, or for a sunlit holiday on some golden sandy beaches of a Caribbean Island. Those foolish thoughts and long gone dreams!

I too thought she was stunning. Hollywood was probably looking for her. This Sister Linda Forester remarkably was our own. She was born in our town, went to our schools and walked on our streets. We wondered how on earth had she got to twenty seven years old and had not been whisked off to Pinewood Studios in London or Hollywood in California and hence become *the Film Star* of our home town. Here, we surmised that her heroine was Florence Nightingale and not Betty Garble or our English, London born, Elizabeth Taylor who had recently finished, 'A Place in the Sun' in 1951. But we still wanted our Linda Forester to be part of 'Hollywood's Golden Age'.

It was not just her looks; she had flair, style and class. She had a walk that future models would imitate walking down the runway in New York, London or Rome. Her Sisters uniform of dark blue and a black cotton belt with a shinning silver buckle accentuated her perfect waist, the lace collar of white was beautifully balanced by her Sisters' cap, which had its edges adorned with an even finer, delicate white lace. Her dress with long sleeves had those unmistakable white starched cuffs, which were actually twice the length of a man's shift cuff. But those cuffs alone suggested authority, and that was an authority she could readily demonstrate.

When she smiled, and she did often, her raw beauty brightened even the darkest of wintry days; her only make-up was the slightest touch of a deep red lipstick. The Casualty Department actually ran a very orderly routine in all of its related departments of the Clinics during the day, with the radiology department, the laboratory, the cast room, the ophthalmic and the psychiatric interview room. Around the corner from the Ambulance Entrance, there were the double doors of the Morgue and its Holding Room that had its own exterior door to the outside. This room was only being used for patients being brought in by ambulance or police, either dead or had no chance of surviving, usually after a massive accident, Casualty also had an Interview Room or Quiet-Room which doubled as a Chapel. Sister Forester kept her Casualty Department and part of the night use Clinic area sparkling. Even from the outside, way beyond the parking area and beyond the first wall of the Fortress came the clear and unmistakable, ever present smell of that overly used disinfectant, Dettol. Dettol 'hung' to the clothing of everyone that worked there. We even imagined taking Linda Forester on an exotic date, to a sunny beach where she wore the tightest of swim suits and even after splashing around on the rolling waves or frothy foam we might still smell Dettol on her, or ourselves, but that was a minute price to pay for a date with our Hollywood Golden Girl.

Each time it became my rotation to work in Casualty, which was always on the late evening/night shift, as it was for all Male Nurses, this night use for the men to work had a secondary motive, safety. Since the Casualty Entrance, as well as the Clinics had frequently open doors to the outside and to a public who may just wander in after seeing our bright shining light above the Casualty announcing what we were to occasional rowdy and drunken people. This shelter from the elements on windy, rain-drenched nights happened quite frequently on Friday and Saturday nights when the local pub closed.

The late night shift meant that I only got to meet Sister Linda Forester at the ending part of my shift. So, in the quieter hours of the night, usually around three am, I began creating a saga of the nights events, from the new babies with stomach upsets, to the acute abdominal pains where an explosive aorta may immediately burst, to the falls from stairs or ladders where broken bones meant sculpting with Plaster of Paris; to the lovely deep cuts from slivers of glass that created open wounds with copious blood flow; to the tragedy of a miscarriage and their sad, unhappy stories. There was, of course, a list of drunken, bruised and black-eyed brawlers late out from a closing local pub, or car-crashed victims cursing 'the other' driver as they howled in pain from low back and neck pain; to the litany of ambulances and police cars bringing in the tossed, tired, tremulous and torn patients or prisoners. I needed these long stories to spend a little time longer sitting next to Sister Forester, here time was not of the essence to go home, but to stay and linger and secretly try to determine which perfume she possibly used today. Perfume was not allowed on the General Wards, but in Casualty, I knew she wore a trace of something exotic!

Every day I thoroughly enjoyed the prospect of giving my report to her, my saga or more correctly, the report of what happened and what I accomplished. The report would be given in her Nursing Office, and she was usually accomplished by her staff nurse, and on rare occasions Doctor William Trevor Adcroft would pop in and add to my story and enlarge upon it, and before he was finished he always said, " *Well done Greenhalgh, lets do it again*", then he would clatter noisily off in his army boots, leaving everyone smiling.

Perhaps it was my bad manners, but those Casualty morning reports I gave, were totally and specifically focused on my 'film star-like' heroine Sister-in-Command, Linda Forester. I know I embellished this nightly tale of high drama, of patients and their injuries with their tales of woe, but with each patient's story, the treatment both 'Doctor Strangelove' and I had delivered so magnificently. It generated a series of questions from her that allowed me to create an impression of my great efforts and skills and my *service to mankind*. Frequently, after ending my report, Sister Forester would make an approving comment and give me that great Hollywood, the true Hollywood Golden Age smile that forever made me her follower.

CHAPTER 7

OB and GYNY

A WORLD OF MYSTERY AND IMAGINATION

Where Death shall have All Dominion

For the Male Nurses, the women's huge Gynecological Ward was a world of no physical Nursing experience. Lectures and wild stories from the two chief Obstetrics and Gynecological surgeons and Consultants had to suffice. There were two senior Gynecological surgeons, both Consultants and both excellent surgeons, Mr. David Marks and Mr. Derek Samuelson, both lectured to us and both told stories that dazzled us in our imagination. However, there was an entrance for us lads to see beyond the hollowed Ward Office of the OB and GYNY Sister. This was Sister Vivian Rivera who ruled here; she always, it seemed to me was constantly gesticulating to men in all manner of male attire to *read the notice and ring the bell before you put one foot into 'My Ward'*. She stressed the word *My* and pointed a rigid finger at the sign.

Our access into this Women's Ward of mystery and imagination was during our training in the Operating Room. Our collective male experience always occurred during our second year of training, and it began very simply. As Male Nurses we were to assist the OR Orderly who would wheel the trolley or stretcher from the Operating Room to the Gynecological Ward for the patient who was next in line for surgery, thereby passing beyond the office of this *battle-ready gatekeeper*, it was all too legitimate and authorized, and we smiled, Sister Rivera would not stop us now.

We were completely adorned in our Operating Room outfits of green, a sloppy hat covering our head almost totally down to our eyebrows, our green oversized gown, that was tied at the back from neck down which opened only the last 12 inches above the tiled floor. But the gown itself almost touched our ankles. Only when we actually had to bend over the bed helping a patient onto the trolley did our baggy green pants show themselves. Below all of this was the white *Wellington Rubber Boots* that kept us electro-statically free. To this identity hiding garb was added the excessively large facemask, but once leaving OR the mask was pulled down below our chin.

Of course, when we were in the operating room during a surgery the mask would be covering all of our face leaving only an inch or two for our eyes. We Male Nurses were the *Bandits of OR* as we called ourselves. Since we *abducted* in a sense, the sometimes-unwilling Lady patients, we felt we deserved the title. To the female Student Nurses of this OB and GYNY Ward we were the *mysterious packages of men*. Their title for us. However, we were never sure if this was a romantic notion or a bewilderment of nothing more than bundles of humanity in baggy clothes. Whilst on the Ward transferring these lady patients onto our trolley to bring them to OR, or even returning them back after surgery, we had a chance to show our lovely sense of humour that actually made us a little bit more *attractive*, well, we hoped.

In this Gynecological/Obstetrics Ward of 36 beds, sometimes overflowing to 40 beds. We wheeled women of every shape and size, from perfect looking bodies to huge rotundas Pickwickian obese women to tiny, frail skin stretched tight over their skeletal body's. Ladies all, but for each person we rolled on to our trolley we had the offered assistance of a Student Female Nurse.

This became our flights of romantic fantasy, even a joy, and a duty to delight in the expectation of what may be. This became, depending on the nurse and her attributes, an opportunity to get body-tight physically next to this lovely lass, as we needed help on one side of our trolley, or the bed from which the patient was coming. We, the OR Orderly and I, could arrange it where the Student Nurse assisting us would have to come so close to us that our bodies were touching as we tugged or rolled or slid the patient onto the trolley. It was a small and an instant temporary reward-Body Contact-to add to our daily journeys. If we were lucky, based on length of operation time, time of day, or this student nurse coming to the end of her shift, we could repeat this *getting to know your body* routine when we brought the patient back after surgery. An extra perk, so to speak, and it seemed like those Nurses did not mind or suspect either?

It was during this my first episode of experience in the OR that I came to the significant conclusion that I did not want ever, ever again to even think about having sex, with the opposite sex. *Sex No!* With all these OB and GYNY patients and that first week in the operating room, so much was new, exciting and sometimes to the point being frightening. Seeing the surgeon place the scalpel on the scrubbed and antiseptically clean bare belly and cut a perfectly straight line from belly-button umbilicus to a spot just above the pubic bone. One fraction of a second a pink skin coloured with an Iodine antiseptic, to the next fraction of a second a bright red cascade as blood vessels being sliced through and pouring blood into the *valley* of flesh the scalpel was creating. Occasionally a fine spurt of blood would shoot up as the scalpel sliced through a small arterial blood vessel and spurted, responding to the beat of the heart. To see it for the first time was a breathtaking, eye-opening miracle that became impaled on my memory receptacles forever. This deliberate intrusion into the body by an instrument so incredibly sharp, swords and daggers were no competition, they were by comparison simply *barbaric blunt tools*, and weapons of ancient history.

The operating room orderly and I had brought this middle aged lady from the Gynecological Ward, placed her on the operating table then after her bare 'ball' shaped belly was prepped and the Anesthesiologist had her completely anesthetized did the Surgeon begin. The 'opening' physician was the House Surgeon who cleansed, sterilized the whole area several times using Iodine, then carefully draped the patients chest, abdomen and legs with large green sterile towels and finally placed a large green towel with its 12 inch square hole in the center. This went directly over the abdomen where the incision would be made. With skin clips each corner was then secured to the abdomen.

Today, Consultant Mr. David Marks was the Surgeon, and masterfully as usual, he made a longitudinal incision, it seemed from one side of her iliac crest-where the hipbone protrudes on one side of the belly to the other side. Probably the precursor to the bikini type incision, but here incisions were incisions, and this was a huge incision. Lots of bleeders, clipped or cauterized, then down through the layers of fat, then muscle and down into the peritoneum, where retractors were placed over this huge open wound that stretched the tissues, then clamped into place, leaving a wide open mysterious cavern. With the exploration incision made I watched the surgeons hand disappear into the gaping hole of abdominal contents, this spectacle I was seeing for the first time and it was staggering, *breathtaking*!

Then Doctor Marks made a decision to enlarge the abdominal access; another larger claw like retractor was placed in the open wound after this smaller retractor was ungraciously removed. The claws working like the fingers of your hand bent to almost touch the ball of the thumb, like a short-legged letter 'U'. The claws spread above and below the incision line and were now gripping the skin and fat tissue with the muscles and peritoneal tissues. The tissues all were retracted and locked into place now giving an enormous open belly of blood tinged organs with globules of yellowish fat tissue and after some of the larger bleeding vessels were tied off, the smaller more prolific blood vessels were cauterized leaving an instant acrid smell of burning flesh. There was constant swabbing away of the blood from bleeding vessels and after irrigations with Saline, both the blood and saline were again suctioned away. Lots of Saline was always used for washing and irrigating the surgical site in all surgeries.

Then to my amazement, visible coming up through this huge cavernous hole a large protruding red balloon shaped mass protruded through the open belly wound.

The Surgeon used the word *'Uterine Anomaly'* describing this bulbous, protruding ball. Whatever it was, to me it looked like a fat, strangely coloured, ugly body part that shouldn't be there; this was my very unscientific observation. How could this enormous Football sized mass possibly grow in anyone and not be noticed before it got to this size?

The surgery progressed and this mass, now described as a *Uterine Cyst* was slowly dissected away from a massive system of support blood vessels and the cob-web strands of peritoneal tissue. Three hours had gone by before we saw how extensive and how immense this cyst was. I had been instructed to bring one of the outsized sterilized stainless steel buckets and place it close to the Surgeon's feet.

The surgeon was bringing the mass of tissue very slowly, yet very surely out of the belly, as it seemed to learn out towards the area between the patient's legs. Finally, the last strands of supporting tissue were separated and this frightening to me, red mass was noisily dropped into the bucket. The bucket was not big enough; the mass protruded another third of its size outside of the bucket! When finally weighed it was twenty-eight pounds of solid tissue. The surgical 'hole' that was left once the cyst was gone looked amazing, the inside of a human body, and looked even more incredible as the surgeon did several more sweeping inspections with his hand. After more saline washes and suctioning, the retractors were removed and a long process of suturing the various levels of tissues began. The surgery and the brief recovery-whilst still in the Operating Room, took a little over five and half hours, almost the whole morning!

This was my first lady patient from the OB and GYNY Ward that put me on the road to wondering if I could really have a healthy relationship with a woman and her lower belly and pubic area ever again–from a romantic point of view-of course, but these real time images can last a lifetime.

The next Gynecological invasion into a woman's body was even more horrifying than my first experience and it happened on Day Two of my Operating Room experience. Today we had Doctor 'Mr.' Derek Samuelson doing the operating list.

At the beginning this second day, I wondered if I would have a gentle excitement to my nervous system, or would it be an on-going easier experience as each day became more familiar? Would a new experience be easier to deal with mentally, emotionally or from a future romantic encounter? I wondered, I was still a virgin and these images in the Operating Room were not what I had ever expected.

Again, Leo the OR tech and I trooped down to the OB and GYNY Ward happily sharing a hope of some *slick-chick* nurse who we could briefly snuggle up to as we slid the waiting patient onto our trolley. But not this time, this patient, barely thirty years old seemed quite agile as she almost bounded on to our trolley. This lady, her name was Grace, was slightly heavier than she should be for her age, and she had been having a long extended and heavy hemorrhaging after having a baby some five weeks ago. Although she seemed energetic her pale face betrayed her low hemoglobin and hence this anemic countenance and body needed a resolution. The resolution for her was, as the Gynecologist had quipped during one of his lectures, the only way was to *look and see* via the familiar D and C. As Students we had learned from Doctor Samuelson that the 'D and C' was the Dilatation and Curettage of the Uterine Canal, done to clear any remaining pieces of tissue, of the Placenta, that had torn and remained attached to the uterus causing the constant bleeding. Then, during that lecture his explanation seemed so academic, so simple to understand, but now the real thing was before me.

Our patient was on the trolley and we were off on our designated journey to the Operating Room; we had picked up her chart at Sisters Vivian Rivera's office where, on rare occasions this *Keeper of the Woman's Ward* when she was not ordering the males species to obey the rules for visiting times and everything else, she would bring the patients' chart to our trolley. In a more caring, gentle even loving voice would kindly encourage the patient on her way to the Operating Room to resolve the mystery of her Gynecological discomforts. Perhaps, and upon meeting the surgeons' knife the possibility of a different diagnosis than the one she had been given when she had first consulted with the Consultant Gynecologist, that always led to a surprise.

Grace, our patients name, had already been pre-operatively medicated on the Ward, and should have been fairly relaxed and sleepy, but she remained quite chatty as we trundled on our short distance to those black rubber doors of the Operating Room, towards the *IN* marked door. One question she asked the Consultant as we arrived in the OR, that totally surprised me being still a little embarrassed with direct sexually related questions-and the visions in the OR. To me it seemed the question she should have asked of her surgeon, long before she climbed on to our trolley, and now she was asking, "I'm going to have a D & C, does that mean after this *'dilatation'* I won't be able to have satisfying sex again because my vagina will be widely dilated"? Great Scot! How do I know, I had never thought about this before! This deserved a satisfying, intellectually truthful and anatomically correct answer. I certainly did not have the answer nor any experience to get even close to an answer! Doctor Mr. Derek Samuelson, the surgeon ready and waiting for this lady, his patient and moving closer to her as we put her on the OR table. He leaned over her and gently and quietly answered her question before she was anesthetized. I had no idea what he said, but I did want to know this seemingly, no *incredibly* important question, I needed to know the answer to this sexually relevant question for my personal knowledge and having that knowledge I could be well informed for any future *female related* questions or discussions. Besides which, who knows what the future romantic relationships were to come in my own life.

Grace, now on the operating table and her legs held up at almost 90º whilst the stirrups were inserted into each side of the table, then her legs were spread and positioned on the stirrup supports. After the sterile-pillowcase-like towels were placed over her legs, Doctor Samuelson quickly draped his patient with the usual large green OR towels over her chest and abdomen. This left the whole perineal area open as the surgical 'site', and as I was the circulating nurse for the Doctor, this was my first time ever to view a widely displayed perineal area. What a sight, oh my goodness! And Thank Goodness for I was under my surgical facemask becoming a bright, beetroot-red colour of a blush that did not stop, my cheeks were burning in embarrassment!

No one had noticed my blushes, because Doctor Samuelson had begun to do lots of swabbing of the whole lower abdominal, pubic and perineal area with Iodine, he moved his stool with his right foot and sat down between the open legs that were held up high in the stirrups. I had placed a sterile bucket between his feet, on the floor. And he began this Dilatation and Curettage. The curettage itself seemed a somewhat brutal action of scraping the uterine wall quite thoroughly to dislodge all the disruptive tissues of the stubborn placental remains leaving a smooth surface. The 'scraping' did cause a fair amount of bleeding, but the hemorrhaging would rapidly slow and usually within 24 hours it will have stopped. Now under anesthesia, and the muscle relaxants working and coursing throughout her body and her muscles, she was completely relaxed. The instruments lined up on the small telescoping table had been wheeled to the right hand side of Doctor Samuelson. Only a few instruments were needed for this procedure but there was what appeared to be a massive odd shaped club. It was spoon-shaped, a shinning stainless steel curved scoop-like ball. No guessing on my part could have quite imagined its actual use. The surgeon gently opening the labia, then spreading the two sides as wide as his fingers would allow then he grasped the *medieval* instrument and with the dexterity of a locksmith inserting the master key into its special place then maneuvered the scoop-like curved end first sideways, then to its intended position where the scoop kept the vagina open as the weighted end hung down between the legs. So, this fascinating sculptured shaped instrument held the *'site'* widely open as would abdominal retractors do the same thing with stretching open the abdominal cavity.

To my continued wonderment, or horror, or both, one vision following the next, the dilation of the uterus began, stainless steel finger like probes opened this bleeding cavity then a slightly larger size probe dilator would follow the last. With the intravenous muscle relaxant drugs, and with the dilators, Doctor Samuelson was satisfied that he had sufficient access to the hemorrhaging interior of the uterus.

My astonishment continued, and with eyes wide open, the next instrument the surgeon used with equal dexterity, as perhaps he had been a swordsman of repute in some earlier life, was with the Curette tool. Besides the one he now held and wielded, other larger curettes lay on the table close to him. This instrument on first examination looked simple enough, a squarish handle with indentations along its four sided shaft, that allowed for a strong and sure grip, and extending from the handle a long round rod which then ended into an open pear-shaped design blade. Its two-sided shape was, perhaps ingenious in its simplicity, since the interior edge was the cutting, shearing, razor sharp scalpel in its own right. This was the Curettage of the 'C' in the D & C.

More anxiety came upon me when the curette was now able to pass into the uterus, and it's seemed as though the whole shaft of the instrument had disappeared from view. It was inside the bleeding cavern of this afflicted womb. It was the tissue known broadly as the *afterbirth*-the placenta-that was being scraped and ripped away from what should be the normal smooth uterus lining. Instead of the placenta coming out as one single mass of tissue, coming out with and attached to the umbilical cord that had been the lifeblood of the growing baby, its detachment was incomplete and the torn pieces were *retained*. This was the culprit for the extended hemorrhaging and abdominal pain and the loss of energy, anxiety, low hemoglobin and sometimes even depression, as well as adding to the possibilities if '*post-partum blues*'.

Once inside the uterus the proof of dexterity of our Surgeon swordsman was evident as he rapidly scraped, explored and cleaned the interior walls of these placental tissue tags. The bleeding was profuse, gushing out coming down and over the spoon shaped scoop of the vaginal dilator and down into that well known and used stainless steel bucket. Satisfied he had removed all the placental tags, he was finished. Doctor Samuelson removed those 'weapons from another age', irrigated then re-swabbed the whole operative area, and stood to leave.

Since I had gone through my first major blushing event. I dared myself to ask the same question his patient had asked, even though I may blush again... So I did, and repeated Grace's question, '*of whether or not the dilation would cause a permanent 'widening or less elastic ability of this vital sex organ'*. Doctor Samuelson smiled knowingly and said, "Under normal circumstances, with average exercising everything will go back to its original healthy position". I was relieved!

He smiled again with that fatherly look of *I know why you are asking that question.* But then he stopped briefly, realizing I was new Student Nurse to the OR so he carefully explained that the procedure was vital to stop the bleeding, if the procedure was not performed the ruptured pieces of tissue of the placenta or the after-birth would continue to erode the uterine wall and at the same time cause the tiny blood vessels to tear and continue hemorrhaging and even become infected. Then he was finished and he was gone.

Was my brain; were my eyes, my emotions and perhaps my rationality ready to accept these visions, these sights and sounds of what the opposite sex actually looked like from a very real up-close and personal point of view? In these moments I didn't think so. What with an incredible football ball plus size uterine fibroid being 'excised' from one woman's sex organs to another whose gaping pubic orifice had instruments of torture placed inside of her, only to increase a torrent of rather badly smelling red blood. Too much, too fast!

There, on the spot I decided *No sexual adventures in my life, end of story.* (No sexual adventures had yet happened, but I was preparing in advance).

Mystery and lots of wild imaginations came upon our Gynecological Ward, and this event ended quite sadly. It was indeed where death appeared very realistically to have *'all dominion'* over these frightening, completely puzzling events.

Over a period of two days, in the darker days of autumn, where day-light seemed only to flitter briefly from breakfast to early tea-time, those late November days were also chilly with cold rain, and blustery wild wind biting into your skin and seemed to smack your face as you realized the wintery snow was at hand, and perhaps to a lonely person, it was becoming a gloomy, depressive time of the year.

Those two days, two separate days a Tuesday and a Wednesday, and between those two days the peace and tranquility of the Ward was separated by a full twelve hours of darkness and stillness that enveloped the Ward and Operating Room. Between those two days a great mystery was unfolding. This fact alone added to the puzzling dilemma of why two women from the Gynecological Ward, died with two days separating their deaths. Both ladies had the same diagnosis and the same surgery; both deaths were totally unexpected, their deaths similarly occurring during the night, neither woman had any complaints, their surgeries lasted the same length of operating time on the OR table. Six other beds separated their beds in the Ward, and the beds were on different sides of the Ward. However, although the Ward staff and OR staff was the same, both women had different surgeons!

Both of these Gynecological patients died post operatively three days after surgery, both showed only brief if no instantly recognizable symptoms! Symptoms would have been classic if we had known the *'infectious invader'* or the flying element carrying their diseases. If these lady patients had had any symptoms, other patients did not observe them from the next beds, or by any staff, or with their family visitors, everything seemed to be progressing normally.

They were admitted into the Gynecological Ward for surgery appearing healthy apart from their Uterine Prolapses, which they had for varying lengths of time. Surgical expectations for even the simplest diagnosis following surgery, as a 'D and C', are for a hospital stay was at least four days. During this particular dreadful time of two patients dying one day after the other, a cloud of gloom set in over every patient, on this Ward patients don't usually die here! The nursing staff had no answers for either themselves or their patients. When the two Gynecological Consultants Mr. David Marks and Mr. Derek Samuelson, the Surgeons or Residents doing their Grand Rounds and a patient who was brave enough to ask the dreaded question of, "How did this happen"? Or "what was the cause of their deaths?" They were simply told the vague notion that an investigation was being conducted. The Medical Staff was at a loss, a profound loss. How to resolve this present medical mystery was of paramount importance!

At the time of the deaths no one could possibly explain their causes. The pathology of two deaths that should not have occurred was going to involve lots of re-history taking, backtracking over physical health and illness, going over and over, and over again. What really happened? How did it happen on two fairly healthy women who simply needed a routine Hysterectomy surgery? Was a wrong drug given intravenously, was an instrument left inside the belly causing rapid decompensating of blood pressure?

Sister Vivian Rivera the Obstetrics and Gynecological Ward Sister went into override with her voice, commands, demands and gesticulations, she was going to solve this crisis if this was the last thing she would do. The Operating Room Sister, Marilla Mitchell though normally softly spoken, became a changed personality. Her face was flushed red, gone was the gentle crimson pink, her voice crackled with anxiety as she meticulously had everyone that was present during those two surgical procedures come back into the OR as we repeated and repeated everything from counting both surgical swabs, surgical towels and of course all the surgical instruments whether used in those particular operations or not. We counted and we searched-searched for a clue to point a finger at the cause of these deaths. The Anesthesiologist checked all of his drugs, recounted his repetitious syringes that sometimes he prepared in advance of a surgery, he checked the drugs he got from the Pharmacy and he called the Drug Companies of the medications he used, related to the same drugs he used on the women. Some one, some-where had to be held accountable, and guilt flooded into the departments that were involved. It was very 'nerve racking', *it was panic*!

Since the Student Nurses did all the housekeeping and cleaning duties in the Operating Room, our techniques for cleaning, sterilizing and then repacking into specific surgical packs were checked for accuracy. The packs were then autoclaved-did they get sterilized? Were needles cleaned and sharpened adequately? Was the red rubber tubing we rinsed constantly for the intravenous administrations irrigated thoroughly then sterilized in the massive sterilizer in the Operating Room? Was the sterilizing time period correct? Questions asked over and over. Answers repeated over and over in each arena of this surgical procedure; lab swabs were taken of the floor, windowsills, surgical tables, anesthesia cylinders, the insides of drawers and door handles, and the swabs went to laboratory for cultures. On it went with a fever pitch to locate a culprit.

Both deaths, in their patient histories had no specific disease nor could a cause be ascertained. The Pathologist carefully looked at these two puzzling deaths, doing post mortems and after searching for a rational explanation by checking charts, lab studies, previous illnesses and family backgrounds gave the rather inadequate title or cause of death as *'Misadventure'*. Misadventure, this unknown cause of a death was used mostly by Coroners who could not determine a reason, even after extensive research find any relevant explanation for the death.

If, by example, a body were pulled out of the local canal, the Coroner would assign the death as, *'Misadventure by drowning'*!

The families of the two women, and a Physician husband of a patient on the Ward at the time of the deaths, demanded of the Hospital Administration a more investigative search. It seemed that we had done our best, and in all honesty it did seem like we had, there was nothing to hide.

Our Hospital Pathologist, an American by birth and education had received his Pathology specialization at Cook County Hospital in Chicago, he simply explained his hometown with the slogan, "It's a really *'The Windy City'*!" (Chicago's nick name) he said in his jovial and happy voice. He was always friendly an expectation we had of those lovely Yanks anyway, the question he had for himself, it seemed, more than to anyone else, was, *'how could the diagnosis, the findings and the conclusion be such an unsatisfactory failure to simply conclude their dual deaths as 'Misadventure',* the quest for truth was still unfinished!

His name was Doctor Phil Ericson III, and we all enjoyed this Americanism of being a third or rather 'the third' sounded very King-like, Royalty from the other side of the pond.

Searching ahead of everyone, Doctor Ericson himself had called to consult with the Senior Pathologist at the Regional Central Hospital in Manchester, and so both had concurred that something was desperately wrong, we were missing something! The two Consultant Gynecologists also had spoken to their respective Chief's of Obstetrics and Gynecology, one at Cambridge University who was on staff at Addenbrooke's Hospital, and the other a Chief at Edinburgh University Hospital and still the answer eluded them all. The provisional verdict of 'Misadventure' for these deaths remained.

It was unreal; it cannot be real! This *Misadventure* category belonged to the death by drowning in the local canal of a person who may have simply fallen into the canals dark flowing water, an accident indeed. These were not our two ladies on two different days, with two different surgeons; no this needed a Medical Sherlock Holmes.

Within six days of the first patient succumbing to a death of mysterious circumstances, we had our Medical Sherlock Holmes in the form of a very quiet fellow with a furrowed brow, wearing a Black Polo Neck Sweater and a Black Suit. He was 'Holmes', so we called Doctor Ericson, our Pathologist his "Doctor Watson'.

This character, a studious, analytical and quiet man held the title of 'Chief of Epidemiology', a Consultant in his own field. Fascinating actually, since he was the lone physician in the whole region, a region that had a University Hospital system and major hospitals for all of the towns within its geographic region, and a huge number of Geriatric and Mental Hospitals, as well as private physician owned Care Clinics.

Within the medical community our 'Man in Black', Doctor John William Duckworth the Consultant Epidemiologist, had two major tasks to perform. The first was that of Professor and Chair of Epidemiology, this naturally included lecturer, teacher and educational advisor to other regional hospitals and as guest speaker at Physician forums. His second position was that of Consultant and prime investigator, a calling that he obviously enjoyed. Previously it was known that he attacked each medical mystery with relish and enthusiasm, and mostly solved those puzzles. From the moment he arrived in our midst, it was clearly understood, that he would stay with us until the question that was on everyone's mind would be resolved with his perfect and precise answer. He was our Sherlock!

Apparently, he began with reading everything that had been written in the doctor's notes, nursing's charting, laboratory requests and results, x-ray findings, as well as notes made by physiotherapists, dietitians – everyone.

All the names of everyone in the charting process were categorized. Others were categorized into those who simply had *direct contact* with each patient, and all others who were indirectly involved both inside and outside the hospital setting.

He wanted relatives from both families to meet with him, and when they did, he wanted detailed movements of where the patient had been, spoken to, had physical contact with, the health of all of these people they met, had any of these people recently returned from overseas? And his notes grew and grew as did his list of people who may offer a clue.

Since Doctor Duckworth had done a Residency in Pathology he was particularly interested in bugs from anywhere in the known world, and in all kinds of bacterial viruses, their classification of kingdom, phylum, class, order, family, genus and species. He considered aerobic and anaerobic species. He wondered about process and the results of toxins, analyzing physical presentations of nervous twitching, muscular spasms, discomfort of skin and mucous membranes-was there discolouration, edema, swelling of legs, face, tongue what temperatures were noted on admission, before surgery and after, time periods involved, was the patient NPO (nothing by mouth), on intravenous fluids or showed signs of dehydration. Did anyone notice any signs of classical or possibly unrelated shock, either neurogenic or hemorrhagic shock, and were the eyes carefully examined. Doctor Duckworth wanted to have the full range of infections and immune epidemiology answered for each patient, before going to the next step. One of his rare responses to the Gynecological Ward Sister Vivian Rivera's questions to him was, "You must always remember Sister, *that every*, yes every process of ill health and disease begin with the *Inflammatory Process* somewhere in our human condition"!

Sister Rivera had remembered this so well, that she had written it down in large letters and made it into a poster, and attached it to her office wall just above her desk. We would never forget its accuracy, this *Inflammatory Process*.

As his investigation continued he had now devoured all of the laboratory findings and so made his way up to the Obstetrics and Gynecological Ward. Here he physically examined each patient's bed, wanting assurances of how each bed was cleaned and how often. He checked the beds for linen and how much there is on each bed, how well the bed sheets are washed – at what temperature of water is used, what soap, and for how long. He went down to the huge Laundry Rooms on the ground flood, watched the washing and drying, then the storage of the linen before it was sent back up to the Wards' Linen Rooms. He examined their linen trolleys and took swabs. Where ever he went he took swabs. He examined the Bed Screens, their wheels for cleanliness or dust, he wanted to know how the patient's meals are served and even spent some time in the Kitchen observing the cooks, utensils and heat of the food processing.

'Sherlock' wanted to know how the patients are moved from the Ward to the Operating Room, who was involved and what process was used. I remember this very well, since our Epidemiologist actually followed the operating room tech and myself from the OR to the Obstetrics and Gynecological Ward, watched us move a patient from the bed to the trolley and so collect the patients' chart from the Ward Sister. This time Sister Rivera was being much better mannered to us than usual, since *she was also being observed* by our own black polo necked sweater-wearing Epidemiologist in a finely tuned quizzical manner. Her good manners appreciated and off we went to the Operating Room.

This *time line* investigation now in progress, we were at the entrance to the Operating Room. Passing through its massive rubber IN door, we were now in the chamber of flying scalpels and other mystical events.

Our Sherlock Homes was all eyes and ears but no words passed his lips. He had previously gone into the OR dressing/changing room and donned the green camouflage cap, shirt, mask, pants and gown, as well as the white rubber Wellington Boots that we all wore, now he looked like one of us.

But no, he was the solitary observer. Obviously he was no stranger to being part of an Operating Room; he knew where to stand to observe both the Anesthesia procedure and the actual process of surgery. He moved away from the table's proximity as an extra-wheeled table of instruments was positioned for the Surgeon or the Nurse assisting with the surgery. He deftly moved away again to the back of the room as the Circulating Nurse brought extra swabs, towels and irrigating solutions. He was a pro. What he was not, was a talker. Each time our Anesthesiologist tried to involve him in a conversation, in either an academic or general interest topic he was met with silence, there was no response, nothing, not even a grunt in reply. This brief exchange between the two physicians that clearly showed who was really in command – and it was not our *'gas passer'* Anesthesiologist Doctor Dennis Holt. Nurses observing this overt 'ignoring of Doctor Holt with a stony silence, seemingly very offensive to him' to the more pompous Anesthesiologist, so further communications ended, at least for now. The Nurses beamed at the rebuff given by one doctor to the other, everything of this nature was enjoyed. A little fun to break up a serious day. One for our side! But who was counting?

Doctor Duckworth watched and made notes as the surgery proceeded. He checked the sterile gloves everyone involved in the actual surgery, he watched the cleansing of the skin, the draping of the towels, the way the instruments were handed to the surgeon and returned back, he watched how the incision was made and how *bleeders* were sutured or cauterized, and how decisions were made about an unseen complication, or how and who chose to do *close-up* of the operative site. His eyes and ears paid exacting attention to everything.

The surgery over, the swabs, towels and instruments all meticulously counted, twice. Then the counts were recorded, as the 'detective' continued his stay with the patient to watch and mentally note the post-operative recovery process. Then he followed the trolley as we pushed the patient's back to her bed. A process repeated several times over during his time of watching how we did our surgeries.

Doctor Duckworth, the Epidemiologist from Manchester, spent two days interviewing the Surgeons their Housemen and Residents; he cross examined the Anesthesiologist, then did the same intensive questioning to the Pharmacist and his assistant verifying to his satisfaction that the deaths were not compromised by any drugs or medications or by a drug reaction.

All the Nursing staff from the Operating Room, from Sister Marilla Mitchell to her Staff Nurses, Student Nurses and Orderly's on both day and night shift. Housekeeping staff had to meet his gaze and questions. After it appeared all the human beings that might be in some way implicated in contact or related services had been completely exhausted did our Man-in-Black', 'Sherlock Holmes' decide to spend the night inside the Operating Room suite, including the changing rooms totally on his own, completely isolated and undisturbed, speaking to no one and so he did, shrouded in the dim lights of OR. He slept there, on the Operating Room table, so he said.

By the end of his sixth day, he came to the simple conclusion that he had to spend a complete day shift and night shift if necessary, in the Operating Room. He arranged with the Gynecological Surgeon Doctor David Marks for him to do an identical surgery as the one performed on the two lady patients who had died.

He was in the OR before most of the staff arrived, he had checked the floor and took swabs to be sure the floor had been completely cleaned with a Carbolic solution and Dettol was used for the furniture. He watched as instruments were unwrapped from the sterile towels that held them and he watched as used instruments were cleaned, scrubbed and placed back in the boiling sterilizers. He noted carefully as patients were brought in placed on the OR table, then their surgical field swabbed with iodine, alcohol then the OR sheets which had a square opening in the center would expose the area to be operated upon. This draping in green towels was done in every instant of surgery; small squares to large square left open for the waiting blade.

From his stainless steel stool in one corner of the OR, he watched, clarified and re-verified! He probably heard nothing, but watched everything.

It was in the late afternoon that the answer came thundering into view. It was a *'eureka moment'*!

Obviously he had been wide awake from the moment he entered this domain, he had watched, carefully noted, re-analyzed, cross-examined the whole arena of the operating room. He had spoken little whilst his attention was on the physical events of the last several days. These intense days in the operating room were all about *observations* to bring a clarity that was missing.

What followed what, or who did what, and how did each action relate to the next action? This time in the late afternoon, his eyes still bright and open, his brain functioning at maximum focus on this afternoon day in Autumn. Through the multi-paneled small glass squares of the only window in the Operating Room high up on the west facing wall, a beam of sun light suddenly shone through the window casting its long beams of light from the window wall across the entire Operating Room to the other wall close to the large black rubberized entrance/exit Doors. As the beams of sunlight had suddenly brought new bright light unto our *'theater of operations'* for a few brief moments it seemed to bring with it a perfect peace, an unusual stillness, a heavenly light, even the timing of a transition where the surgery had just been completed and the final surgical dressing had been applied.

Our Sherlock Holmes, who had been sitting on a stainless steel stool in close proximity to the larger of the two bubbling sterilizers-it was warmer there, suddenly screamed at the top of his voice, *"Stop everything and speedily place another larger green towel over the patient"*!

Surprised, no one had the foggiest idea what was happening. The Surgeon who had come running back into the Operating Room half dressed from the changing room after hearing the word *'STOP'*, fearing some cardiac emergency or even a massive hemorrhage, yelled *"What, what"*? The remaining five of us in various tasks of the post operative cleanup and restocking was simply stunned into dead silence.

Being sterile in this moment of time and space had no meaning. All our eyes were on 'Sherlock' our Doctor John William Duckworth our Consultant Epidemiologist thinking that he had either cracked mentally or more hopefully had miraculously cracked open the mystery. He was standing at the side of the Operating Table, with both hands stretched over the new clean sterile towel, which had been placed over the patient at his command. He was preventing anyone from removing the towel. His eyes and head riveting from the green towel below his outstretched hands to the highest point on the ceiling directly above him, this action of looking down then up again lasted for several minutes, and no one spoke. Then, he asked everyone not to speak, so our trance-like positions remained, even the Anesthesiologist who was still in the process of bringing back the patient to a sleepy consciousness was for the first time quiet. The Surgeon who had rushed in thinking the worst for his patient had also resisted a massive temptation to question his Epidemiologist colleague who had raised his right index finger to silence him, even after his original anxiety of 'what, what'.

Was this a magical, mystical epidemiological moment? Ready for this record-making event to be recorded in the mighty annuls of medical practice?

And then he spoke, *"I'm almost there"*, he said. He then had one person on each side of the OR table, hold the towel with out-stretched arms-which had been covering the patient, hold the sheet high above the patient and move very slowly to one side which would allow the patient trolley to be moved in, the patient carefully moved from the OR table to the trolley and out of the OR back to bed. The two people holding the stretched green towel then moved back over the table and laid down the towel spreading it over the OR table.

During this extended moment in time, the sunbeams of light were gone, and the usual incandescent lighting surrounded us, but the huge OR light above the table was still on. Doctor Duckworth thanked us all for our quiet patience and told us he *'thinks'* he has a probable answer to the deaths of these two Gynecological patients, but more time was necessary. The answer would still be many hours away. The Surgeon left puzzled with his questions still unanswered. The Anesthesiologist asked the questions for all of us. "What did you see or perhaps conclude that would make you shout out *'Stop'* and frighten us all to death"? Doctor Duckworth answered this question simply by asking another question. *"When the sun flooded the operating room with those bright rays of sunshine, did anyone see anything, anything?"* The 'anything' obviously was becoming connected to what had caused his outburst of *'stop everything'.* No one had seen or heard anything. Finally, now began the investigation that would enlighten the world of our aging, presently guilty Fortress-like Hospital.

Doctor Duckworth, from his seat on the stainless steel stool had instantly been aware of the bright sunrays coming into the operating room from the window on that west wall. What was particularly of interest to him and unseen by anyone else was a sparkle, a brief flashing star-like tiny piece of stardust, or debris as it passed through the bright shaft of sunlight. The sunlight, almost unreal in itself on this wintery Autumn day, this shaft of starlight, broken by a twinkling particle of something floating down as light as a tiny feather, passing through the sunlight and on down to rest upon the green towel covering the operating table. How could this speck of mystery be the cause of so much havoc and death?

Doctor Duckworth very slowly and very carefully wrapped up the large green towel that had, maybe, become the repository of this tiny, sparkling piece of debris or dust, or a simple flying element, and he wanted that speck!

Even though it was late in the day, where staff members were already going home, Doctor Duckworth's demand for an instant Administrative meeting was quickly called which included the Gynecological Surgeons, Pathologist, Medical Consultants, Administrative and Senior Nursing staff of OR and Gyny. Doctor Duckworth wanted to close the Operating Room until he had thoroughly examined the ceiling and its natural composition – the paint, plaster and even the woodwork behind the plaster. He wanted no further surgeries until he was finished even if it required a week or more to do it! With Public Health Services behind him no one argued, Operations were rescheduled and other Hospitals within our region notified that they might get some of our intended patients.

That night, whilst the ladders and scaffolding were being set up for him to have easy access to the ceiling, he spent over four hours, he told us, with a magnifying glass trying to find the first piece of ceiling, the tiny fragment, or a dust particle that had dropped from its ceiling perch. He found nothing; the green sheet had either lost this speck of evidence or camouflaged it within the fabric, his first fragment of evidence was not to be found! That night he went to bed a renewed man, besides which he would be sleeping in a real bed! Now he was more eager for the new day to dawn so that he could focus entirely on his precise methodology, a new day of discovery to explore and tear away the ceiling!

He knew what he was looking for. Once again there was no sight of his black polo neck sweater or his black suit for he was dressed in OR greens and he was alone apart from the Orderly and myself, in the Theatre. Climbing up the ladders to the safely secured platform, then lying on his back on the platform he maneuvered into place. Once he had reached the center of the platform he placed all the jars that had screw-on lids that he brought up with him, within easy reach of his arms. At this point on the platform his face was less than 15" from highest point of the ceiling directly above the operating table. Although the table had been moved he had marked the position where an *'open belly'* would be in relationship to the highest point of the ceiling-where he was now.

Now his early morning orders to get both of the large sterilizers coming up to the boiling and to keep the water boiling were in full power. The steam silently billowed up towards the ceiling, and his perch. It was my role as Student Nurse to be his assistant that fascinating day; to keep an eye on the sterilizers and be available should our 'building inspector' Epidemiologist need anything. Our American Pathologist Doctor Phil Ericson III popped into the OR to watch progress occasionally and ask if he could help.

Once Doctor Duckworth had reached his perch, with a variety of trowels, chisels, forceps and his several glass jars; as well as green towels, which he laid at arm's length away from him. Now he said he was comfortable and expectant. He wanted to lie in his chosen position looking up at the ceiling, until the steam from the sterilizers accumulated at this zenith of the ceiling, which he now more clearly recognized as the highest point of the ceiling itself, the very gentle slope of the ceiling from this highest peak was not noticeable from the floor, it simply appeared more flat.

Within half an hour and propping his head on a few towels for support he seemed satisfied with his first conclusions, and as the steam created a thin veil of vaporous cloud, and before he began to scrape he pulled his face-mask over his nose and mouth. The steam coated plaster was collected in the first glass jar and after more scraping the powdery plaster quickly filled the jar and then other jars. He had exposed about an eighteen inches square area, which was directly above the center part of the operating table. At this point he took a break and came down from his lofty, steamy perch bringing his filled glass jars, then he marked the jars from the beginning and in order.

After forty minutes of enjoying a cup of Darjeeling Tea, exercising his arms and legs, and gathering more empty glass jars, back up to his Crows Nest in the OR. The next layer was much thicker, perhaps an inch thick. This layer was easier to scrape, more porous and crisscrossed with a fine fibrous membrane or rough cotton-like thread. This cement-like lime, a grayish white plaster when scraped away came down in small clumps, rather than the powdery dust of the first layer.

Small clumps of this plaster went into the glass jars, as did larger pieces filling four of the larger glass jars, again in order. Beyond this layer was a more heavy and fibrous layer, where strips of wood could be easily seen, and between the wood strips lying length way's there appeared to be what looked like *straw*. Certainly a common natural product from any farm our field, economical but here? The remaining jars were filled with this packing or insulation of straw and the jar lids tightly closed. This whole deconstruction of the ceiling had taken almost five hours. And our scientific investigator had been lying in this back for most of this entire time. I had been off for lunch and returned, and so when he finally told me he was satisfied, I could not help wondering if he would have developed 'scaffold sores' on his whole back from lying in one position for so long. If he did, he never told us and I never asked him.

Now, with this glass jars placed in two boxes he took them down to the Pathology Laboratory, and refused my help to carry the boxes full of jars, he wanted complete control of his ceiling specimens, and untouched by anyone else.

He was exhausted and looked it, dark rings almost surrounded his eyes, and so he wisely announced he was going back to his hotel to sleep and refresh his brain.

A newly washed, bright and beaming, hair combed, white lab coated Doctor Duckworth, wearing his black polo neck sweater, arrived in our Dining Room for early breakfast and from all reports of our only waitress, who normally only served in the Doctors Section of the dining room she had reported he was the first person to arrive for breakfast, sat in the first chair of the first table that he came to (this table was the table assigned to the lowly First Year Nurses), but he was hungry and ready to explore his glass jars.

Before he had finished breakfast he has been surrounded by first year students coming for early breakfast themselves, and they were amazed that their Guest-by now the talk to the entire hospital staff, would chose their table. A small banter of conversation ensued between them, since he was energized to get downstairs to the path lab and begin his microscopic investigations. Apparently he did tell these nurses that he would let them know once he was sure of his findings. He promised them a lecture on his approach to Epidemiology, and why he thought he had the possible answer to the two deaths.

The operating room remained closed, and most of the staff was reassigned. Surgeons grew anxious and sent the more urgent surgical emergencies to the towns other hospital. The Administrators, desperately wanting the exact cause of death of our two patients to perhaps punish or admonish-someone! Wanting too, to get the operating room repaired and repainted or whatever was necessary to get back to full capacity. In our Fortress Hospital there was a gleam, an air of expectancy that was noticed by everyone. We all wanted the magic of the moment when Doctor Duckworth would say, *"It's done, and I have the answer"*!

Three days later, after he had finished scraping the moist ceiling, he had the incredible answer; but not until the fourth day after he had called, then brought to our hospital another Senior Pathologist from the University of Cambridge. Holding the mighty position of the 'Chair of Pathology' this Physician came and consulted, and together they went over 'Sherlock Holmes's' meticulous findings and conclusions. They did concur totally, with no doubts.

The deaths, both deaths were due to Tetanus.

Tetanus! The medical staff was amazed and totally puzzled. How on earth had this Tetanus Toxin, this poison so deadly, have been introduced into our hospital? Or, like a silent assassin coming into our operating room unseen, unknown, leaving us all unaware of its presumed dead or attenuated form. No one could bring in and place so precisely a bug of this historic character of darker days. There it was, proof positive, this wretched killer had done its worse.

Doctor Duckworth, our Sherlock revealed his insight; his presumptions, and his clinical findings, it was amazing. The Fortress Hospital had been built a couple of hundred years or so earlier, and it had gone through several changes and renovations. All the corridors had remained unchanged but the rooms and halls of various sizes had been redesigned for many different uses many times. The Operating Room suite and its adjoining rooms had been chosen carefully for easy access to the main corridor and the larger high ceiling room that, with only slight remodeling became the Operating Room. The huge circular, operating reflective light had been suspended on the only cross beam high in the ceiling. The peak of the ceiling where the steam from the huge sterilizers collected was two feet away from the cross beam; however, it was at the highest point or the ceiling from which our suspected invaders floated down to precisely the point of an open abdominal wound on the operating table and sliding over the big OR light, to the waiting open wound for this flying element of disaster.

At some point the original, or a later renovation of the ceiling, which must have been done more than one hundred and twenty years ago according to all available records, it was common practice to use horse hair mixed in with the plaster which gave the plaster a better 'holding' or adhesive character. The tetanus spore had long before attached itself to one of these hairs, Doctor Duckworth knew this, and because in his painstaking examination of all of the material he had scraped away he found two other spores firmly attached to hairs. As the steam accumulated in that specific area of the ceiling it created sufficient warm and moisture to decay the layers of plaster. In turn a hair or two also decaying released the tetanus spores that fell through the weakened plaster and so finally glide slowly down into an open waiting abdominal wound. Its unseen, unnoticed passage had even avoided by being irrigated away with a final saline solution wash. Long surgeries required a saline irrigation-and suctioning at each layer, as the open wound was being closed and ligated back together. Remarkable that the Tetanus Spore, *only in these two instances*, had clung to the inside of those wounds creating such disaster.

Both autopsies later revealed the same cause of death, Tetanus Toxoid Poisoning. This cleaver and adaptive little fellow, the Tetanus spore is one of those rare bacteria that can live in a 'attenuated' condition for a vast number of years, more correctly its name is Clostridium Tetani. This attenuated bacteria is able to diminish its size, surround itself with a fat like membrane, and then hibernate till an opportune time comes along. It needs an environment without oxygen, so its termed 'Anaerobic', it needs a lovely warm body 97º-99º temperature of a human being and preferably in a closed off part of the body where the constant body heat can warm up the outer membrane and so dissolve its fat like layer were its Toxins are then released into the blood stream, and most often, this kind host- us, we die!

Doctor Duckworth kept his promise to the Nursing Staff, and invited all the Nurses to attend his lecture. It was a grand illustrated lecture and presentation about the Anaerobic invaders that can kill us or give us a nasty dilemma like 'Lock Jaw'-a symptom of Tetanus poisoning. He shared some aspects of his intensive search with us that went unnoticed otherwise. He had been to the local Library and the City Council's Planning Department to check local farm-lands, illnesses of families and farm workers; he checked on the building construction of our Fortress and changes that may have been recorded.

In his lecture, he spoke of the tetanus spore being warmly wrapped up in human tissue not requiring oxygen to survive. This anaerobic organism wants to become fully alive at normal human body temperature. The spores are found throughout the world in the soil, animals in their teeth or faeces carry them, they are found on Horses hair, on dead grass or crop remains. Even dirty instruments like knives, scissors or needles may carry this spore. Any cut or skin breakdown can harbor this aggressor! This spore may have been in its previous state for the last hundred years or more, being attenuated, or 'asleep'. But in the dark and at 98.4` hibernating is over! So begins its desecration of the host. In our Operating Room both the ladies who died, had a sad misfortune of being in the wrong place, at the wrong time. The question arose, of course, why did not more people become contaminated who had been having surgery on the operating room table? Always when there was surgery, the sterilizers were both 'on' producing lots steam, over the same time period as the ladies, either before, between or after them, so why not more Tetanus problems? A variety of answers were offered but the truth remains a mystery. As long as we get vaccinated with Tetanus Toxoid we have a fine safety web around us, was his advice.

Doctor John William Duckworth's recommendations were approved, a new sub-ceiling was created and the sterilizers were moved to an adjoining room. Yes, death here had *'All Dominion'* and its events were indelibly emblazoned on all of us, but the Truth had been discovered.

CHAPTER 8

ORTHOPAEDIC'S

CHISELLING BONES, ROMANTIC MANOVERES, A NIGHT AT THE FLICKS

The Orthopedic Ward, with its Male and Female Wards to each side of the Fortress Hospitals' Main Corridor always seemed so very lop-sided, because there were twice as many Female beds as Male beds. Now, for myself as a Male Nurse, and equally for all the other Male Nurses, we really enjoyed this disproportion of patient sexes, especially since we were constantly in demand on the Female Ward. We were needed for a variety of duties from making beds, lifting patients in and out of bed, assisting with the re-application of plaster casts and the joy of it all, being a support for a lady needing to be up out of bed for walking exercises. These wonderful tasks were made much more exciting when the patient was anywhere between sixteen and thirty six years old. When this was the case, help from the Male Ward came instantly. Well, almost instantly, if we were helping one of our male patients get in or out of bed we could quickly find a reason to postpone that duty for the *emergency need* to go to the Female Ward to assist.

There was always a prospect of a romance there. The only inter-ference with this romantic agenda was when the patient we were helping on the Male Ward had his lovely daughter visiting or there was a small group of female friends and visitors at this man's side. Then we had a voluminous number of reasons why we needed to stay at this man's bedside. Generally this ploy worked well with the younger girls, those under twenty five, we never seemed to fail at getting them to be *grateful to us* for allowing them to visit. This veiled deception we used in the evening when the Ward Sister had left for the day. Visiting Time rules only allowed two people at the bedside at any one time. So if our dear old patient had three or four visitors and two or three of them were young ladies. I would, like the other male nurses, always be firm in my conversation about visiting times and number of visitors. This got me to the bedside and the focus of everyone's attention, and a lovely conversation about number of visitors by capitulating to their requests to let them stay, I was in theory anyway, would be in great trouble by allowing them, especially if the Sister were to return and find that I had disobeyed the visiting rules. The likelihood of the Ward sister returning was almost zero but I did get their combined gratitude and comments of *'Oh, you're so kind; or 'you're so nice and oh how sweet you are'*! Sounded like Hero worship to me, how great we are. What joy it was to be in a position of power like this? This Orthopedic Ward was the place to be, no blood or guts, just infections from time to time. No sudden death or bouts of deep paroxysms of desperate coughing that brought up the green globs of phlegm. This was *'Nursing'* of a different degree, this is what I had mysteriously signed up for, and this was a resplendent calling for mankind. Romance was in the air the possibilities were beginning to seem endless. The Orthopedic Ward was on our Nursing Rotation for each of our three years. Could anything be better than this? Romance had to be here somewhere, the young lady visitors on the Male Ward and the young lady patients who needed our physical contact on the Female Ward. For Testosterone, much lives here.

The Sister for the Orthopedic Ward was somewhat temperamental in nature, with that long thin face and pointed chin, she wore too heavy glasses that constantly slipped down her nose and she had a voice that was high pitched and seemed to have a razor sharp edge to it when she became annoyed or anxious. So don't make her anxious! Fortunately this did not happen often.

This and the fact that she was tiny in stature, only four feet ten inches tall but with her nursing cap which she kept folded and creased at two inches taller than it was meant to be, gave her an odd 'telephone pole' appearance, especially when she had her rapidly graying hair wrapped up in a tight bun which oddly balanced her Nursing Sister's cap. But she did have a gentle loving streak in her and when she smiled her face changed with a pink blush colouring her checks. She was certainly authoritative, and knew how to demand a fine quality of Nursing Care, where she would on occasions come and help doing whatever needed to be done-doing a complex dressing, removing sutures or even helping make beds. From that point of view she was a rare Sister. She was kind in so many ways that with her forty two years old mannerisms all the Nursing Students would like to give her a good passing grade.

I too, liked this Sister. Her name was Geraldine Jones and I liked her from a very biased point of view. Three years before coming to be a Nursing Cadet at the hospital I had been a patient on this same Orthopedic Ward on two separate occasions over an eighteen-month period. Everything that had happened during those days of surgery on my left arm, I remembered quite clearly, and Sister Jones had treated me with gentleness and caring reassurance like I might have been her son! She had welcomed me on my arrival in the Ward, and during the days of preoperative preparation before the surgery, she came to my bedside and asked if I needed anything. Upon waking from the Sodium Pentothal anesthesia induced sleep, she was there again letting me know that everything was good and I was back in bed and safe. Post operatively she took a little extra time to ask how my arm felt, and did I need any pain medication, and spoke to me each day of her patient-to-patient rounds prior to the Consultant Surgeon coming in to do his Pre and Post Surgical rounds. Sister Jones had been good to me, her patient, and now I was on her Ward as an up and coming Nurse!

The Orthopedic Consulting Surgeon, losing his official title of Doctor, like all other Consultants was Max Colgan, M.D. This fine Physician, Mr. Colgan was the finest dresser of all of our consultants, if you were to see him for the first time, anywhere and unannounced, you probably would have guessed he was at the pinnacle of his profession. He was five foot, ten inches tall, with a round pleasant face adorned with a generous, but well manicured moustache. His fair, almost blond hair was plastered flat against his head. His hands stretching out of the extended cuffs of the sparking white shirt and he had beautifully sculptured hands and fingernails. His cuff links, always noticeable, gleamed no matter how dull the light may be. Mr. Colgan always, and for all events, wore an elegantly tailored pinstriped suit, in a usually dark navy blue colour, and he had a full-buttoned waistcoat to match. Out of his left breast pocket elegantly protruded a three cornered, two-tone purple silk handkerchief and it was always at the exact same position coming out of his pocket. His patent fine Italian leather black shoes, shone with perfect ebony black and the soles were leather. He also announced his approach by the sound of his hard leather soles clipping on the hospital's tiled corridor floor. His brisk walk creating a long rapid drum roll as he traversed the corridors.

Much like other physicians his age, he too had been in the Royal Army Medical Corps. Before going into the Army he had completed his Residency in Orthopedics, and so served as Orthopedic Surgeon in the RAMC. Mr. Colgan, had he been wearing a military uniform now he would likely have been a Colonel. In keeping with his military career his time keeping was precise to the second. When he wrote orders they had perfect clarity, just as his voice portrayed a clear, understandable certainty. Of particular importance for his patients was that he was a good listener and he could direct or redirect his patients, who frequently wanted to give him their life story, back to the pertinent issues of their present pain, discomfort and anxiety.

Consultant Mr. Colgan was the perfect antithesis of our uniquely bizarre General Surgical Consultant Mr. David Peter Alexander. These two incredibly gifted surgeons could not be more alike from all their dress mannerisms, appearances and colourful characteristics. Even to their dining habits and their cars, Mr. Colgan car was always immaculately polished and sparkling clean, where our Surgical physicians car was coated in grime, mud and would have had snow thickly laden on its top and bonnet-had it stayed cold, apart from that window wiper area, which only the window stayed relatively clean.

It was Mr. Colgan who had correctly identified the cause, given a diagnosis, and recommended an instant resolution to the increasingly painful lower left arm of mine-that was being treated as a 'sprain' for three months by a general practitioner. This 'pro-tem' Physician, standing in for our General Practitioner the Family Doctor, was less versed in the finer art of correct diagnosis. His instant resolution to my parents worrying about my pain, was, "Your son has simply sprained his arm so take him back home and put a firm bandage on it".

To my fourteen-year-old brain the treatment I was receiving from him this GP seemed completely wrong. But he was the Doctor and in those days there was no arguing with the Doctor he was always *'right'*. It was not until the dark hours of any early morning in January, when snow had been falling since dinnertime and was still coming down filing up on pathways and roads, that the pain was becoming so intense in my whole left arm, especially above my wrist, I could find no position, or exercise or even a really tighter bandage to give this excruciating pain any relief. I had to freeze my arm and there was only one way to do it!

Clothed in cotton pajamas and a dressing gown only covering my right side, I couldn't use my fingers to tie the gown so I came down the stairs, opened the doorway to the bitter cold of the night air, then over short pathway to lie by the side of the streets gutter where the icy water was flowing on towards the drainage hole. Lying in the snow with my arm completely immersed in this really icy water of the streets gutter, my arm rapidly numbed and the pain lessened! It was cold but the pain was momentarily gone.

After ten minutes, I think, I don't remember how long, my father came out dressed only in his pajamas and he was frantic, *"What on earth are you doing,"* and "Why are you in the snow, and in the street- *and why are you half naked"*? So many obvious questions, and he half carried me back unto the house. He was fearful for me on various levels, but realizing my pain was so intense and there were no medications, only a silly bandage to help the falsely diagnosed pain as a sprain. My Dad Eric had to initiate some action, and at daybreak we were on the bus to the Casualty department.

An x-ray was done and read quickly at the hospital and an urgent consultation made for me to see the Orthopedic Surgeon Max Colgan.

From Casualty we went across town to Mr. Colgan's Surgery, where he made me his first patient of the day. He retook more X-rays of the Left Radius, Ulnar and hand bones, then, in a quietly spoken voice told my parents that I had Acute Osteomyelitis with a Brodie's Abscess in the bone marrow. The increasing and unremitting pain was caused by the swelling from the inside of the bone, and since the bone contains the 'bone marrow' the solid bony surround-ings make any pressure that builds up inside the bone becoming extremely painful. This difficult and emergent problem requires the immediate opening of the bone, then scraping and cleaning away of the very infectious abscess.

"Here is what I want you to do", he said, "Take him to the hos-pital today and I will do surgery in three days. The Brodie's Abscess in the lower part of the Radius Bone, needs to be drained and removed" and I will see him tomorrow in the hospital as he is being prepared for surgery".

Off we went to the Hospital Fortress, and my world began to change. That is where I met Sister Geraldine Jones, and my bed in the Orthopedic Ward.

In three days I was on my way to Surgery. My Orthopedic Surgeon, Mr. Colgan did exactly what he said he would do-he opened the bone with a Stainless Steel Hammer and a finely bladed Chisel. Then scraped and chiseled away the infected marrow, then cleaned the bone and surgical area, irrigated and swabbed it dry. Finally, the remaining marrow and bone was insufflated with Sulphonamide Antibiotic powder, and it healed. Unfortunately, in one way, this first surgery had to be repeated almost a year later since the pain and its intensity had returned. The second surgery was successful but did require more bone tissue being chiseled away, and leaving a permanent indentation in my left wrist.

Fortunately in another way, I became a lot more familiar with this Ward and Staff!

In order to get an accurate History and Physical of my disease process, Mr. Colgan questioned all possible events that would have led up to the reason for the Osteomyelitis and Brodie's Abscess. He summarized that, during a football match for my school team, as a defending left full back, I had been confronted by a player intending to beat me to the ball, and although I got to the ball and cleared it first, I instantly knew that my opponents right boot was aimed at my poor old unprotected scrotum, and his boot was coming into region very fast. My instantaneous reaction was to put my left arm and hand out to protect my 'future heritage', so instead of my scrotum being pulverized my left wrist was injured and badly bruised. No bleeding on the outside. That was the moment of impact from a dirty boot, Mr. Colgan believed, that a miserable Staphylococcal Bacteria entered my arm through a tiny unnoticed cut in the skin, and since the Brodie's Abscess was directly over my *foot balling injured arm*, that was the best logical explanation.

It was these adventures of my own surgeries that brought me into the inner sanctum of the Fortress Hospital, and so began a healthy fascination of a myriad of questions and the mysteries they held.

It was a good decision since the remainder of my professional life would be working in hospitals across the world. A decision I would happily choose again.

This Orthopedic Ward was enjoyable in so many ways as a Student Nurse. First, second and third year's Ward experiences more than compensated for the acute pain and misery of that Osteomyelitis and its two surgeries that followed. The two five-inch scars on my left forearm, became a 'medal' of sorts from my early athletics, besides which, our school team made it to the finals for two years running, winning each Final and so earning that prestigious, gleaming trophy.

As a Student Nurse on my first year's rotation through the Orthopedic Ward, it was the Staff Nurse who held all the power and authority for the Ward in Sister Jones' absence. This lady in her own right was a well-endowed beauty, quite voluptuous with curves in all the right places and in perfect proportion. She was pretty, probably in her early thirties, and always had her raven black hair cascading equally over each side of her round face and it seemed that her dark brown eyes under superbly shaped and her cultivated eyebrows, glittered. There was only a gentle touch of colouring from a light red lipstick and when she smiled those lips appeared to quiver. But who would even notice, and I was only gauging her beauty from a purely 'artistic' point of view.

This was Staff Nurse Jane Brandwood. Who, besides being a beauty in a uniform was a gentle mannered, never ruffled by anything, very communicative charge nurse. Actually, it was only on some rare instance that either the Ward Sister or her Staff Nurse would have to discipline anyone, and that discipline always came in the form of a teaching moment. Staff Jane Brandwood had an obvious-the number of finely suited fellows visiting her- and an *envious* list of admiring men both young and old, but her heart appeared to have been won by this Resident Orthopedic Surgeon who was in his last year of Residency at our hospital. None of the Male Nurses liked this character, nor did I; we thought he was too slick, too smooth and too pretentious, to be an honest to goodness suitor for our Staff Nurse Jane. We all believed she was just mesmerized by his amorous advances.

When they met, which were several times a day, and every day they were both on duty, he never failed to touch her body somewhere. The *'somewhere'* was generally around her waist but occasionally his hands reached below her trim waist onto her bottom. These were supposedly surreptitious and momentarily brief flirtatious brushing by each other whilst on duty. But all could see.

Perhaps we were at trifle jealous! I know it was more than that; we wanted a gentleman, a man of strength, someone who was dark and debonair, a secret agent kind of character. We wanted a man who could treat our lovely lady with more gentleness, and more respectfully, than this flirtatious Orthopedic Resident. A man who could show others how well he could love rather than maul a woman.

I know we were all unimpressed by Doctor Brian Christopher Melanie's desire to look into the mirror in the nursing office, and constantly check his overgrown wavy black hair, patting it down to make sure no hair was out of harmony with the rest of his wavy hair.

He would check his teeth by clenching them tight together, opening his lips and with his little finger of the right hand, dig between his teeth to dislodge some offending particle of food. We judged him to very proud of his face even to be enamored by his own looks. *"Oh, you handsome devil, you"*! We would mock him unkindly.

Doctor Brian Christopher Melanie was fortunately born to wealthy parents in Pathos, Greece. From there they had moved to Hanover in Germany, and then moved again to finally settle in West Looe, in Cornwall. He had taken four extra years at the Universities of London and Oxford to finalize his medical degrees, now here he was as our Senior Orthopedic Resident. Here he was, it seemed to be more interested in his amorous pursuit of our Staff Jane Brandwood than on coming to the Ward when we needed him.

Whenever she was on duty, day or evening shift, he was there presenting his attributes of smiling, open mouthed, perfectly aligned and cleanly picked teeth. Generally he would gesticulate with wide and high arches of his arms and hands allowing one of his hands to briefly touch the uniform of our Jane, our Staff Nurse, these gestures, noticed by everyone were simply seen as pathetic overt overtures of desperate romance. But what was more astounding to the other male observers was that Staff Nurse Jane actually responded to this blatant Romeo's sly connection to her uniform—with demure smiles as she turned her body toward him, in public no less!

On the days when Staff Nurse Jane was on duty, and even on the days when the Ward Sister was also on duty, it usually indicated that both sides of the Orthopedic Ward was full, and also that there was a fairly lengthy list of Orthopedic operations still in progress, or alternatively, that patients on the Operating List had extensive surgeries that could last for many hours. On these days of lengthy lists or long surgeries, we knew that amorous Doctor Brian Christopher would not be coming to the Ward until quite late evening and Staff Nurse Jane may have left duty for home especially if she had started work at seven am. So when Doctor Brian Christopher did arrive on the Ward he would be spending the next period of time doing his post operative rounds with me, or one of the other male nurses. Strike one for protocol, for the lads! No Romance here.

During my second year's rotation to this great Orthopedic Ward, Doctor Brian Christopher and Staff Nurse Jane had become engaged. Both were in their mid-thirties of course had every right to chose each other, but the entire staff would have chosen different and opposite partners for them both.

This, unapproved event by the staff, created more angst for all of us, Staff Nurse Jane now worked more late shifts, coming in at one pm and thereby not leaving until ten thirty pm, it was an unusual shift probably to accommodate the *'Love Birds'*. It was also arranged, that Doctor Brian Christopher, had been assigned to Late Orthopedic Clinic when there was no OR Orthopedic surgeries, so this arrangement had him going a full day sometimes going until eight or nine pm. From the Clinic he would come up to the Ortho Ward, take his Staff Nurse fiancé to dinner. They both returned together to spend more intimate time in the Nursing Office-if we did not need either one of them. In the Office they were not totally isolated even with the door closed, the glass pane in the top half of the door gave us all an opportunity for brief quizzical look inside the office as we passed by the door, and we passed by the door more often than we needed, checking on the Love Birds. To make sure they were still there!

There were occasions when we as Students needed to use the telephone to call a patients relative or the Pharmacy or Lab, then we had no option but to interrupt these 'resident romantics', there was only one telephone in each Ward, and it was always in the Sister's Nursing Office, so we had to make sure at least two or three patients needed to call their homes. This was a bit deliberately unkind, but we did it with so much finesse, Shakespeare would have been proud of our acting talents.

It had also become clearer of how both Doctor Brian Christopher and Staff Nurse Jane had been able to 'convince' our Ward Sister Geraldine Jones of the necessity of scheduling Staff Nurse Jane to this later shift.

It was from an ongoing, deliberate and very cleverly conceived bribery. Doctor Brian Christopher's parents lived in West Looe a wonderful, cozy coastal village in a picture perfect cove where once upon a time pirates lived here and sailed their galleons in an out of this almost concealed seafarers Port. Looe looks out into the Atlantic where the whole world's oceans ebb and flow. One of Looe's delicacies was delicious Cornish pastries, but even more than that is the world renown Devonshire Cream that Doctor Brian Christopher brought back with him after visiting his parents, and the happy, delighted recipient of all these trips with the resultant Devonshire Cream was Sister Geraldine Jones. She probably would have vacated her office for these romantics at the drop of another extra offering of this fresh and most delicious clotted cream.

Night Shift on this Ward was wonderful, that is, after Doctor Melanie and his amore' Jane Brandwood had left for home, and all the patients were medicated with either their postop medications or their routine pain and sleeping pills. Visitors from family members to physicians all gone home, then it was 'lights out', that is apart from the small table light of very low wattage that always stayed on the small center table in the middle of the Ward where the Night Nurse sat with a cup of coffee or tea, extra flashlight, and Nursing Notes to be composed.

Since the Orthopedic Men's Ward was much smaller in the number of beds than the Female side, in fact much smaller than all the other Male Wards, it was really easy to track the sleeping patterns their breathing sounds and other noises. There was, of course the occasional bout of coughing, or snoring or even someone talking in their sleep, but once we Nurses became familiar with the rhythm of the night and the free or labored breathing patterns, it all became routine. If the Ward was full, which was frequently, there would be no 'outside' interruptions of new admissions, and rarely did an operation go into late evening. This occurred generally because the patient who had been in the operating room earlier in the day having extensive spinal, hip or femur repair had developed secondary hemorrhaging and had to be rushed back to surgery. This usually meant that there was no peace in the Ward until the patient returned.

On days, evenings or nights on this Orthopedic Ward, only rarely did a death occur, so the breathing rhythm of a body in its last moments, that sad stertorous, noisy rattling sound of lungs fighting to find any tiny measure of oxygen, as life's battle was being lost.

On this Ward it rarely ever happened, so instead we could listen to a story of someone talking in his sleep, or more remarkably practice hypnosis on sleeping patients. I practiced this hypnotic process of standing at the foot of the bed and repeated over and over quietly, "You need to urinate now, get up". Occasionally it seemed to work, but who really knows, perhaps it was just the normal call of nature!

Should the eventuality happen-of a dying heart-on this Ward, either Male or Female nurses would jump to that dramatic, though the Female Nurses believed it barbaric, the practice of making a speedy determination that their patient had stopped breathing and with no discernible pulse, Carotid or Femoral Arteries, as well as swiftly placed stethoscope over the heart, showing no response of the heart sounds. Then we would spring into action, filling our 20 cc. glass syringe with two ampoules of Coramine, the cardiac muscle stimulant, place a three inch Spinal Needle on the syringe then plunging it into the space between the ribs over the heart. The plunge with this lance-like surgical weapon went deep into the heart muscle and we pumped in the cardiac wonder drug, the *Needle in the Heart* routine!

This was the grand final act of medicine *and* Nursing by those magnificent 'Knights in white coats, the Nursing Students!

So it was, here on this more peaceful hospital Ward that life as a Student Nurse seemed to be a perfect setting for taking full advantage of our role as a modern Florence Nightingale. It did not matter that she was indeed an incredible Lady, for we were like Medical Monks! As sleep enveloped the patients, we found time to wander over to the Female Ward to check out which lovely lass was working, so on the pretense of offering whatever help they may need; of course hoping that they needed help like, getting some young lady out of the bed to do walking exercise-in the middle of the night, but we tried. The idea of *helping* was always the best way to begin a conversation, and quite often we were asked to help. It was possible that whoever we were helping would lean in towards us for support, thereby hanging on to our waist or shoulder. Well, it worked every now and again, and if we were scheduled several nights together with the same Student Nurse, the more the better since we could look forward to a *'lean on me'* experience once again.

It was here on this Orthopedic Ward, on my second year rotation that my first romantic relationship began. Sadly, I was not the one to initiate the romance, and I remember a quiver of guilt about my manhood, since I should have asked for the date first! Knowing that I did not make the first move, and later realizing I was not experienced or well learned in high romance-that, indeed, everything about romantic ideas was *all talk for me and my friends*! This conclusion was so imprinted on my consciousness that it became a guiding principle in my future romantic adventures. Ask first; make the first move, its more masculine, testosterone driven and I would be choosing the right person, wild or otherwise!

Her name was Claire Whittam, and she was a third year Student Nurse. It seemed remarkable that she had gone to the same Junior School that I had, although she was only one year older that I, I should have remembered her, but my memory of her remained blank, although I tried so hard to place her face, I could not, she was somewhat of a mystery, and that's why I said, *"Yes"* rather too quickly. I may have had an ideal beauty carved into my literary understandings of pure delightful, and perfect beauty. I Loved poetry, and reading the old classics; besides which, my father throughout his life, recited love poems of the Romantic Poets to my mother, always finding time to lyrically tell her... *"Love is not Love, Which alters when it alteration finds...If this be error and upon me proved, I never writ, nor no man ever loved", or " She walks in beauty", or " Shall I compare thee..."*

Wonderful memories of how to woe and keep a woman! Well, I thought.

So upon my innocent life enters third year Student Nurse Claire, and she had come from the Female side of the Orthopedic Ward. She came so quietly I did not hear her footsteps; she came in stocking feet, not wearing shoes. I was sitting at our small table in the middle of the Ward with the low light shining on the charts, where I was doing my first entry charting.

Claire did not say a word, but made her intimate presence known by touching my left elbow against her thigh. Her thigh! The pressure of our bodies touching was a magical, nerve twitching and a shivering event. Certainly not accidental; a touch of excitement from somewhere within me tickled my brain and brought an unusual sensitivity from this meeting of bodies in the darkened night hours of the Orthopedic Ward-surrounded by patients. Was this the beginning of passion? Was this maneuver a pressure to arousal? From Claire, there was no, 'I'm sorry', instead a whispered statement of, "I first saw you when you came into the Obstetrics Ward with the operating room trolley to pick up one of the patients, and even though you seemed to be in a hurry, I saw your eyes and those long eyelashes of yours. They are lovely you know, and I decided that I needed to get to know you much better", she continued, "you were all dressed in the operating room garb, with your green gown and that silly OR hat that is always too big, but your mask was pulled down under your chin, so I saw the face that had those dark brown eyes and gorgeous eyelashes!" I may have said, *"Oh really, well I'm glad you think so"*. This was my introduction to Student Nurse Claire Whittam as I shivered in excitement, she was now rubbing my back and shoulders, this has to be the beginning of an affair I thought, what else could it be? I believe I could even smell her body fragrance, those pheromones that are distinctively personal. We chatted for awhile, and I discovered she now lived on the other side of town very close to my dear uncle and aunt, that she was an only child and that when she finally graduates as an R.N., she wanted to be a Captain in the Royal Army Medical Corps. Before we parted, actually we were interrupted by one of my patients asking for pain medicine, we made a date and arrangements to go the 'flicks' the movies, the next Saturday night, and so we said our goodbyes, I was both excited and quite anxious!

I could hardly wait. I shared my midnight encounter with my friend on the Surgical Ward; he eagerly listened and wanted a moment-by-moment report of our date when we next met. We were both about the same age and probably equally illiterate in the ways of sex, passion and romantic twists and turns, so our talk was cheap. It was hard to wait those four days till we met on Saturday evening, I remembered stories I had heard from the lads older than I, and I remember reading the wild secret meetings of the Gardener in 'Lady Chatterley's Lover' but do I remember the how, why and when to respond to each nuisance of words and the more important touches. In truth, I had no experience of any past sexual adventures or any sexual anything's. I was still a virgin! No past sexual adventures. At this age of my life I was unlearned and totally inexperienced in real romance. My only reference points were reading the weekly magazine, that renowned Tit-Bits' but that was just a silly gossip newspaper with great photos and listening to older chaps brag about their conquests.

All I had of everything romantic seemed much too little to meet the basic requirements of a full-blown encounter with an experienced woman. Everyday till that evening I thought about it, and everyday I became nervous.

Finally came Saturday evening, and so came Claire. We met at the entrance to the film theatre; it was called the Palace Cinema. She looked exotic more lovely than I had remembered her from that *'night of her thigh'*. Even though it was a cold November, quite a wintry night, she wore a short coat barely at mid thigh, and it made her look quite sexy. Was this short skirt an introduction to what was to come I wondered? Her face seemed flushed, radiant, happy to see me as I was to see her, we held hands briefly before going inside but she squeezed my hand tightly, was this a message or simply that my hands were cold and her hands were quite warm, was she sweating I wondered. I was, it was a cold sweat! This was my date, I happily paid our entrance fee so we could sit at the back of the cinema, and since we were quite early for the show we got to sit at the back and in the middle of the back row. Like the fine gentleman that I was trying to be, I helped her off with her coat. Another shiver of excitement overpowered my body, realizing she was wearing a flimsy blouse through which I could see the outlines of her bra, which obviously held ample bursting breasts. Oh, yes, I had seen many breasts, bellies, thighs and pubic hair on women of all ages on the operating room table-and were frightened by some of them; but here and now this was different story altogether, and this body moved miraculously towards me, again. Was this body being offered to me before we had even sat down? Even more important, could I handle this enormously precious gift of a young man finally becoming a man of experience, a man who would and could share this exotic romance to my fellow colleagues at some future, distant day?

The film began and our bodies moved closer, much closer, since there where no arm rests separating the seats we really could get *'hot body'* close. As the lights dimmed, and the film played on, our interest had migrated from the moving pictures before our eyes to the movement of our hands and arms, our lips met and noises ensued, kissing noises perhaps even cooing, I was losing track of my emotions, our arms locked and we pulled each other closer, now I could feel her breasts pressing into my chest, and my shirt was opened as she pulled me closer yet again. These moments seemed to last an age of there own, it was hot and I felt sweaty and steamy. I could feel a bead or two of sweat rolling down my spine and giving me shivers. What's next and how do we do it, do what in the cinema? My mind was racing to keep up with the emotions rolling over me in waves. It was confusing, puzzling, sweaty!

Then, like another profound physical reaction her hand was on my thigh, squeezing my leg, releasing the squeeze and repeating the process methodically. Her hand moved up to the crotch of my leg, 'great heavens' I managed to think could we do this in the cinema with people of both sides of us. She must have felt my sense of uneasiness for now she pulled her coat over both our knees and thighs. This was to be the camouflage of a more erotic exchange that was to be performed. Her hand moved over the buttons area of my pants and my manhood must have been noticeable. If she touches my hardened manhood I might just explode on the spot and be incredibly embarrassed. I must have been close to exploding-but I was also beginning to feel very uncomfortably; perhaps I was squirming trying to find room in my pants to decrease the pressure of these now tight pants. But suddenly her hand released my leg as she dragged her fingers slowly back towards my knee, first explosive crisis was over! Now she simply held on to my arm with both her hands and leaning over whispered into my ear as I felt her moist lips on my ear saying, "Later, when you take me home". So we watched the remaining part of the film without much interest. But the pressure on my arm from her did not cease. The film over, my nostrils full of her pheromones and her perfume still lingered, as we walked to her home. I don't remember the walk, but I do remember the ensuing events of failure! It was a cold night, we held each other close as we journeyed towards her home, and we did not notice that wintry, chilly night.

Her home was one of the groups of terraced houses that had the front of the home facing the cobbled street, and at the rear was the backyard with its door, and the doors opened onto the 'backs '. This back passage way for all of the homes was an unpaved narrow pathway wide enough to allow the rubbish truck to pass up or down passing all the back yard doors of all the homes. From the door there was usually two steps down to the unpaved back. It was to these two steps that our journey was to end-but I did not know it!

We got to her home, to the back door and she climbed on to the higher of the two steps as I stood facing her, and so I was below her reaching up to kiss her. This was, it seemed awkward for me, my arms reaching up to be around her waist-for balance as much as anything else; as she deliberately moved my arms lower to be around her bottom, but I began to fall off that second small step. She must have been quite adept at this maneuver, for as she pulled off my over coat I shivered with the instant chill, she then asked me to help her take off her coat, I did and she shivered, now with both our coasts off and our lips touching, her hands were way ahead of even my thoughts, how could that be? But her blouse and bra were off even before I recognized the brazen action. I could feel her breasts now moving 'to and fro' across my naked chest. This was yet another erotic sensation I had never felt before-was it so evident that I was totally unschooled in this sexual process? Well, yes, of course it was, and this was just the beginning! All of my how's, all of my can I's, all of my realizations that this was the moment that all my adolescent dreams, imaginings and even secret ideations of looking at photos of scantily clad maidens on some exotic beach, or lounging provocatively over the railings of a swimming pool. Well this moment was to be the culmination of those dreams, a Grand Finale of sorts, as I obviously now felt I was stumbling into the romantic 'stud' I thought I should be!

Stumbling was Claire Whittam too! She was in command of the moves, the sounds, and the advances the majestic maneuver on that back step. The whole 'comic opera' she probably thought later, her almost naked body seemed like a contortion as she moved up and down from side to side as she tried desperately to get my pants open and down, but she probably realized that I was not just a virgin to be defrocked but I was actually fighting against her advances by deliberately moving into positions that would make it very difficult to get my pants off! Was I mad? Here was a nymph in the night, offering all her glorious attributes of lust and love-I never knew which, and here I was avoiding this final contact of sweaty, panting man-woman explosions. Claire had moved from the top step to the bottom step to get a better angle of attack, and I, perhaps as numbly switched to opposites steps; then we would both be on the same step. We were gyrating together but my efforts to keep my virginity must have been wearing her out, not in exhaustion but in shear exasperation with me. Finally the moment was over. She quickly gathered her shed clothing, after putting on her coat and jamming panties and bra and whatever else into the coat pockets, she opened the back yard door and disappeared inside.

It was a long cold walk home for me; perhaps I deserved it. No words of 'goodbye' in fact, whenever we met again in the hospital she never spoke to me again!

Indeed this 'first encounter' and its memories lasted a long time into my future, but perhaps as a self preservation mechanism I always recalled the events with a sense of humour so did my close friends, where they laughed and joked at my expense. For a while when either seeing Claire in one of the Wards or corridors or even recalling that night, I could feel my cheeks becoming quite warm as I blushed a deep red. All this began on the Orthopedic Ward, this same Ward where I either admired or had a sense of jealousy of the resident lovebirds Doctor Brian Christopher Melanie and his amore, his fiancé Staff Nurse Jane Brandwood. Well, now I recognized that 'real' relationships required Love!

At some point of this nursing career of mine, I knew there must be another hot romance to come, unless my failed romantic night with nurse Claire Whittam had been shared with all the other female nurses, and if that was the case, I was sunk as a romantic date or conqueror or as a reliable partner, my days might be over, but hope upon hope, those old romantic poets did mention 'love lost,' or was it, 'unrequited love'? I would have to refer back to *'Love is not Love which alters...'* Oh, Shakespeare where are art thou now?

CHAPTER 9

The PEDS, Pediatrics

The Shed of Tears, and Unimagined Beauty

The building closest to the Nurses Home that housed only those lovely female Student Nurses was the Pediatric Ward. The building itself was originally created as two prefabricated 'sheds' or office buildings but was now cleverly reinvented, refurbished and reintroduced as the Acute Pediatric Ward and the Education Building, (these buildings were actually smaller than the Hospital Wards).

Pediatrics was divided into two 'Peds' Wards, where the hospitalized children were placed into age groupings rather than diagnosis or critical nature of a disease. It worked well and there was a good space between all the bassinettes for new born, cribs or cots for the children up to three years old; and the other side for all children up to twelve years of age. All the children faced towards the center of the Ward similarly to the other hospital Wards. There was a small table that during the day held a huge plastic 'smiling clown', which at night became our charting desk with its low electrical light. The Sister's Office was the first office encountered coming into the vestibule entrance from outside. Here there was no veranda to take cover under during bad weather, so if you were coming from Casualty, the Nurses Home or the main Fortress Hospital you simply braved the weather.

Sister Office was perfectly placed both close to the entrance and at the angle of the two Wards. This gave her, or whoever was in the Office, full vision of who was coming and going, a distinct advantage since there were windows from the office looking out onto the walkway to the PEDS Ward, as well as windows overlooking the two main sections of the inside of the Ward. The room next to the Sisters Office had a partition that divided this room into cabinet's of instruments, drawers of medications, and shelves of medications in bottles. There were bottles for liquid meds, bottles for pills and tablets, ampoules of injectable medications in storage bottles, bottles of sterile water, bottles holding narcotic medications or the sterile water vials to mix or dilute the powered meds, and glass bottles of various sizes of intravenous fluids. It was a miniature Pharmacy and all the Third Year Student Nurses prepared and administered those medications. On the other side of the partition were the dressings of every size and shape of various materials. There were bandages, Elastoplast's, splints and crutches of various sizes and colour. In the room opposite this medicine room, was our 'clean dressings' room, it was also where we had three different sized sterilizers, which were always bubbling with boiling water and bursting with clouds of steam. The large sterilizer used for the stainless steel bedpans, urinals and the kidney shaped dishes, then two smaller sterilizers for needles and syringes in one and surgical instruments in the other. These were forceps from mosquito size to the larger sponge-holding forceps, there were tiny 'butterfly' suture scissors to the heavy scissors used for cutting away plaster casts; there were scalpel handles each designed to take a wider straight or curved general cutting blade. It was probably very fortunate throughout the hospital that the Male Nurses tasks of sharpening the tips of all the needles, subcutaneous to spinal needles that we did not regrind the delicate and intensely critical surgical blades. New ones were used each time. Never the less, the Male Nurses were masters of the perfect stiletto fine points of all needles. They were swords in our hands, craftsmen of the weapon and swordsman in their use, we could become journeyman Blacksmiths if necessary! Send us into any battle and we could get that needle into any arm, buttock, arteries, veins or the heart! Plunging in perfect accuracy, none would dare call us foe!

Pediatric Ward was lovingly cared for by a rotund, bursting at the perfectly ironed white apron buttons, as well as the white reinforced cotton belt that was pulled far too tight around her middle. The belt created an unkind, uneven hourglass figure that must have been uncomfortable, even difficult to breath in. However, her Sister's nursing cap of distinctive authority was frequently left in her office rather than on her head. I asked her on one occasion, when the Matron was coming on her weekly rounds, checking on staff and greeting the children, if I could go and get her Sisters' cap from her office, she said simply, "No, my children knock it off more times than I can count, and Matron knows my story about that silly decoration." This Sister was no ordinary firebrand! I knew this lady held a power to be reckoned with.

This was Sister Sandra Desmondhalgh; she was truly a gentle, beautiful soul. When she smiled, her lovely plump rosy red checks seemed to quiver. Her voice was soothing, tender and when a crisis loomed there was an unquestionable reassurance, a hope not yet recognized. Sister Desmondhalgh was the only sister that actually gave lectures to the Student Nurses, and she insisted that if the Ward Orderlies had completed that portion of their work they too should come to her lecture. She had a gift of teaching, everyone from Staff, Parents and Children, as well as a remarkable ability to talk to these babies and children of all ages. Occasionally where there were two or more boys, recovering after surgery on the Ward who became noisy and rowdy. Perhaps unmanageable for a less experienced nurse, but she could bring the boys to instant 'behavior modification', where silence and even good manners reigned again! I loved this Sister; she was another example of a true Nurse. This fine Lady with all these lovely attributes of a real Florence Nightingale, it seemed she encompassed everything that was essential to be a nurse! Her Staff Nurse was Jennifer Foxhouse, who, in physical characteristics was an opposite of Sister Desmondhalgh. She was slim and her attributes for being a professional model seemed in perfect place. Her long golden hair, shoulder length and perfectly straight, but when wearing her Staff Nurse Cap, those long tresses were neatly styled into a tight bun, however, when working with the children-off came her Cap. Whether her hair was hidden in a bun or cascading towards her shoulders, her long elegant oval shaped face had a radiance and natural beauty filled with confidence. She had bright blue eyes that shone with an intellectual understanding of those little people who resided on her Pediatric Ward. Jennifer Foxhouse she was good too. She had the knack of getting an intravenous needle into an unseen vein even in the tiniest of newborns. The eccentric, yet quirky, Doctor Keith Varley, our Pediatrician, taught this unique skill to her. It was he, like some of his fellow consultants that were the *'inner soul'* of this huge meandering institution. They were the teaching staff and part of the inspiration of this Hospital, that perhaps we unkindly called it, the Fortress. These men were not in medicine to make a fortune, nor to make a famous name for them-selves, for they were here on behalf of a genuine human desire to heal and serve mankind, or in Doctor Varley's case to heal these tiny tots.

Doctor Varley's innate skills appeared endless to me. He was a great communicator, so whether listening to him in the classroom setting or doing his own patient 'Grand Rounds' on Pediatrics, he explained everything in a very clear understandable language, and when doing a teaching moment of a pediatric disease process to overly anxious parents, he was exceptional. He innately understood with crystal clarity when a critically ill baby was losing its battle for life; he outlined the changing physiological actions in the child's life systems, how each body organ functioned inter-relatedly with all the others, he detailed laboratory reports with the parents leading to a changing diagnosis and therefore, a prognosis. Doctor Varley meticulously went over all the pro and cons of using a new or different drug, or the need for a further, more specialized consultation, or having the child moved to another research related hospital, he always wanted the ultimate best for *'his'* children! When all treatment modalities had been ruled out and his little patients' had only hours yet to live, he would be there at the crib or bedside with the child, the parents, brothers and sisters or other loving family relatives, and he too would shed tears of sadness. A greater sadness born out of his own disability that he could not have saved this little life; the child could have been his own, even his only child for which he did his utmost!

As a diagnostician, Doctor Varley was the Master of Masters. Although he carried a stethoscope dangling out of his back pants pocket, he rarely used it, which seemed odd to me, but I was just learning about his Pediatric wizardry. He, like our other master eccentrics, was an absolute scholar of utilizing our own God-Given senses. It seemed he could hear and see more than others, a child's barely audible crackly wheeze when breathing or crying; the rebounding noise of an empty belly-but infected from a per-forated appendix or gut; when tapping with the index finger of his right hand upon the out stretched fingers of his left hand that were lying on a very painful abdomen—the solid thud or the hollow pitch coming back from his tapping, would lead to an accurate diag-nosis. His fingers touched skin, and the moist, dry, feverish, or tense skin related a physiological change from normal that he accurately interpreted. Doctor Varley's nose too, could smell all of the dif-ferent odors of skin or other body odors; even the smell of a new-born's faeces or urine had its own healthy or unhealthy odor. These nuances escaped others less experienced. His eyes never missed changes in pupil dilation or contraction, his gaze noticed changes in fingers, hand or toe movement, in a more pronounced walking gate where brain activity may be suspect, and he noticed the tiniest of nervous tremors. All these sensory attributes he put to superb use, since babies who could not communicate, except by crying, grimacing and smiling, or simply being at peace. He simply had a rare gift, and he used it.

It was his skill with spinal needles that made him a specialized 'Spinal Tapper' so much so that other physicians asked him to do their difficult spinal 'taps'. To see him put a baby in the correct posi-tion to be held by a nurse while he found the perfect space between the vertebrae then, using the smallest of spinal needles, with lots of iodine, he could find the precise spinal cord spaces and withdraw the telltale Cerebrospinal fluid. Whist I was there, he never failed with this duty. He could find the spinal fluid the first time, and this technique alone was probably priceless!

He only did these Spinal Taps after much soul searching, since he recognized that whenever there was an invasion of the body's surface tissues, there was always a possibility for an infection, and *that* he did not want, ever!

When lecturing to us in the classroom, he would frequently arrive late. I don't think it was because he was tardy, but more for effect. He would stroll into the classroom with an opened umbrella-even when it wasn't raining outside. He wore a Deerstalker Hat, much like the hat Sherlock Holmes would wear with the front brim of the hat was pulled low over his forehead, an air of mystery perhaps? Between his lips, his teeth tightly clenched on the end of a long stemmed, classic Meerschaum Pipe. This pipe, a lovely instrument with the carving of a Reindeer on its bowl, may have had tobacco in it, but it was never lit or smoked, However it was used to exaggerate an important point during his lecture when he would raise his arm, grasping the pipe and pointing at some imaginary illustration, then quickly lowered it as if to bang it on some unseen desk. Under his tutorship, there was much to learn. He would give us, *his* Student Nurses, every opportunity to ask questions either about the lecture just given or about any of the critically ill children we had on the Ward. More often than not he would go well overtime on our lecture period, particularly if the subject touched on his 'sensory perception' ideas of gauging a child's progress. Doctor Varley spoke with excitement, vigor and enthusiasm becoming very animated while walking between all the student's desks, occasionally even banging on some of them! Often his topic would recall a piece of historical medical mystery, which he would relish with its colourful explanations. Grand Rounds with him, which began every morning at 7am, before he went to do the clinic, or a rare home visit, were always eventful. Sometimes his humour with the children was brilliant. He, similarly to Sister Sandra Desmondhalgh and Staff Nurse Jennifer Foxhouse could get a smile, a giggle or genuine laugh out of these hurting children; this was a joy in itself. Always after his Pediatric Clinic had ended he would return to the Peds Ward and, if necessary, would even interrupt his Clinic if needed back on the Ward. When called to come back, he never argued with the Sister or the Staff Nurse he instinctively trusted their judgments.

There was always much to see and learn from our Consultant about the varying diagnosis, or surgical interventions, some requiring strict isolation, some were referred to us as 'mysteries' from their Family Practitioners, to be investigated by Doctor Varley, who always and carefully arrived at an accurate diagnosis. Only on rare occasions would he call in for further recommendations or an actual consultation from a University Pediatrics fellow or researcher. There was only one occasion I remember him calling upon a Tropical Disease specialist when he was dealing with a child who had recently come from the Far East with the parents who had been 'up country' in a tropical forest for several years.

It was during my third rotation through Pediatrics, after I had my two days off, when I came on to the Ward and learned that a new baby patient was being transferred in from a much smaller hospital on the county border. The five-month-old baby had been hospitalized there since its birth and due to the baby's lack of progress, required specialized neurological care. Since Doctor Varley was regarded as well-known Consultant of Pediatric Neurology, he happily accepted this child. Before the baby was due to arrive, he called his 'Baby team', as he referred to all the Nursing Staff of 'his' Pediatric Ward including the Peds Department and Clinic to a meeting. Doctor Varley wanted to discuss this Baby's diagnosis and prognosis, and how he intended to proceed with treatment for this particular baby, with the baby's diagnosis more careful nursing procedures were required. I had been chosen as the team leader and the baby's nurse, of this I felt very honoured. My third year nursing skills on Peds were becoming recognized as a reliable and capable in every aspect. I loved and thoroughly enjoyed everything about my job, from observation to delivery of care, and the responsibility of decision-making. Then, I was given the key leadership of the second and first year nurses under my wing. I was ready. Doctor Varley had relied on me for reports on many previous occasions, so I knew his trust of me was considerable. I believed in in this Physician's utmost skill, and masterful grasp of treating these little ones. I considered his judgment absolute and his ethics beyond compare.

The 'Baby Team' assembled in Sister Sandra Desmonhalgh's office and Doctor Varley introduced us to our task. The baby's name was Anne Lancaster, and at five months old she *was* developing 'normally' except for the life-threatening abnormality of a slowly growing *Spinal Anomaly*, which we learned was a Spina Bifida! Doctor Varley explained Baby Anne's dilemma to us as a sad set of circumstances that develop 'in uterus-in the embryonic state,' as the baby slowly grows. The vertebrae bones of the spinal column begin to form and provide the vital protection of the spinal cord, in Spina Bifida some vertebrae do not completely form and close correctly. This in turn allows the Spinal Cord to protrude through the open vertebrae and form a 'sac' frequently filling with CSF, Cerebral Spinal Fluid. The nerves, coming down from the brain that give our body its unique ability to move from the movement of our shoulders, the fine movements of our fingers, the use our legs to find balance and walk or how we do our daily activities of living from urinating to responding to pin pricks. Nerves flow from the brain forming the spinal cord, and the cord is protected inside an elongated balloon-like membrane that is filled with cerebral spinal fluid. This fluid actually surrounds the brain tissue as well as the delicate spinal cord. This is a brilliant function. The fluid literary bathes the brain and cord removing any particulate matter, and hence there is a constant flow of spinal fluid at a specific pressure. Unfortunately, in Spina bifida the membranes under greater pressure of the fluid, push the surrounding covering membranes between the still open bones of the vertebrae and so the cord tissue herniates through the spine, which begins to form a significant bulge on the baby's back. The bulge is filled with spinal fluid and depending on the size of this bulging anomaly at birth, could possibly be a major disaster. Especially if this occurs with a woman who is a 'prime-ip', having her first baby, and during a rough delivery process, the pressure in the birth canal can be tortuous. In some circumstances, the bulging membrane may herniate further, which could possibly rupture and so end the baby's life. In those days of long ago there were no Ultrasounds to alert the Gynecologist of a developing Spina Bifida.

Doctor Varley laid out his treatment plan after his overview of the baby's Spina Bifida. At birth, Baby Anne had only a barely protruding herniated bulge, perhaps just over an inch at birth, big enough; her mother was 'multip' having three previous successful healthy deliveries prior to Baby Anne. Generally this indicated that Baby Anne's delivery was relatively easy and the without complications, which it was.

Wisely, the delivering Obstetrician had called in the local Pediatrician who recommended the baby stay in hospital so the bulge could be 'watched' for a few weeks. Those weeks had grown into five months and so had the size of the bulging hernia grown. Now the size of this Spina Bifida extended just over three and a half inches from the skin surface of the baby's back.

The parents were increasingly becoming very distraught. The Nursery nursing staff who was caring for the baby also continued to push the best they could for the Pediatrician to contact a Neonatal Neurologist. Their caring for the baby presented problems like positioning in the crib, nutrition, exercise and even playtime. Further, which medications might be helpful and what possibilities were there for a surgical removal of this very real death trap? To all outward appearances, Baby Anne seemed at peace, she was not fidgety nor did she appear to be in any discomfort or pain. She was a pretty baby, and apart from this growing Spina Bifida, she seemed to be perfect!

Finally, the baby's Pediatrician contacted the right Neonatologist-Doctor Varley and so, without further discussion, the transfer was to be made the same day. So we waited for Baby Anne to arrive. She didn't arrive as expected; her parents had second thoughts about sending their baby so very far away from where they lived and since they had three other children, visiting their Baby Anne would be difficult at best. But after lengthy family discussions and a talk with their vicar from church, they finally, but sadly agreed. Doctor Varley, Sister and Staff Nurse had already left for the day, so I would be the Admitting Nurse, which was appropriate, since I was also the nurse assigned to her care. The ambulance arrived with our Baby Anne and even before the child was brought into the PED's Ward I had called Doctor Varley so he could return back to our Ward.

Baby Anne was wrapped in those lovely soft woolen blankets and surrounded by pillows; she had the most beautiful features of a baby I had ever seen. Her face was that of a Cherub. A sculpting by Michael Angelo, this was the face that would launch a thousand ships in some far away land. I did not know a face as lovely this could belong to a five-month-old baby, but there she was, and she was my baby to care for and love. In this baby's face was perhaps the face of God, a creation of heaven and earth and I was responsible for her physical needs, my heart and perhaps my soul were already prepared for all she may want. Since her parents would only be able to visit on Saturdays I would become both her Dad and Mum... at least to the very best of my ability.

Doctor Varley arrived shortly after we had settled Baby Anne into our Ward. In this part of the Ward there were three other babies under two years old, so at times it was a noisy little corner with crying babies wanting more baby formula or pediatric pain medicine. Doctor Varley, hearing one of the crying babies went over to its cot before coming to see our newest arrival, Baby Anne. His hypnotic coo's or musical magical sounds to the crying baby worked and within minutes the baby was peaceful; he wanted a time of quiet to examine our new baby.

Now began the exhaustive examination, starting with the baby's head to check neck for rigidity and flexibility, then her eyes for equal or unequal dilation of pupils, as well as rapidity of eyes to follow hand motion moving from right to left. For this Doctor Varley used a fluffy, multicoloured small doll, and always Baby Anne's eyes followed his hand movements. He was specifically checking for brain function via the optic nerve, the third major cranial nerve coming out of the brain that gives us a look 'inside' the brain. The optic nerve and its reaction give a basis for the brain's general health or other disease processes. Here, pupils reacting equally or differently on each side versus the other, and pupils not reacting to light by contracting then dilating as the light moves away, great indicators.

Doctor Varley looked into Baby Anne's ears, nose and then with a tongue depressor, into the mouth and throat. He listened to her breathing and tickled her so he could assess how well she filled her lungs, as she gulped for air. He began the palpation of her abdomen; he smelled her diaper so he could determine how well the kidneys were filtrating her urine. On her diaper too were some fresh soft faeces, so he smelled again, making an assessment of her bile duct and the gall bladder's production of bile; as well as how well the intestines and bowel were processing the baby formula and pureed apple sauce. Arms were rotated, and extended, as were legs; he used his reflex hammer on elbows and knees and ankles. He pinched the baby's skin, pressed on tiny fingernails and checked the instantly blanched colour returning to show a good circulatory system. Lastly, he used the handle of his reflex hammer to draw a line down the soles of these tiny feet to check on nerve function from spine to the body's extremity.

Satisfied with this preliminary examination, we both turned the baby over, where I held her cradling her in my arms so that the Doctor could have full access to examine her spine and its awful bubble-like growth. With delicate gloved fingers he held this sac, filled with life giving spinal fluid and gently moved his fingers around the skin from which the protrusion extended. He shone a bright flashlight into the surface of the sac on one side as he observed the opposite side to see how much light might be reflected through the sac and its fluid, or if, perhaps there was a smaller mass deep within the sac. Finally, from his small black bag he pulled out a set of delicate calipers. The calipers had been especially made for him of plastic, made by the leading manufacturer of surgical instru-ments, so he knew that its measurements were precise. With the calipers he measured the bulging Spina Bifida from three separate angles from its forming circumference; and whilst the baby was in an upright position with my arms supporting her body, he also measured her head. These measurements were vitally important in noting progress of the size of the Spina Bifida, or a further complica-tion of Hydrocephalus developing, but more hopefully, a reduction in size of the spinal bulge. During this whole physical examination of Baby Anne, we heard only a brief gentle whisper escape her lips, but no crying or apparent discomfort. Perhaps the warmth of being held or being in an upright position for an extended period of time was soothing for her.

The physical exam and measurements now complete we laid her down again on her side. It was to be our constant treatment modality for her to keep the pressure of her body weight off that protruding ugly bulge, so we moved her constantly from side to side. This was important to make sure she did not develop any pressure sore on either side of her otherwise perfect body.

This unfortunate child was such a good baby, eating and sleeping well, she looked angelic lying at peace in her cot. The next two months I spent a lot of time caring for Baby Anne. Her parents came to visit faithfully once a week on Saturday afternoons. I enjoyed talking with them, letting them know how well we cared for their youngest daughter, but my heart was growing heavier both for them and for my little patient. Doctor Varley was measuring the Spina Bifida's size every few days and with each new measurement, an increase in size was noted. To my eye, I could not see any daily changes that he measured, but by the end of the second month, there was indeed an increase in its size, it *was* growing larger. The following Saturday, Doctor Varley scheduled a conference with both parents again. He had two proposals. First, was to consult with the leading Pediatric Neurosurgeon who two years previously had written a thorough review of Brain and Spinal Cord Anomalies in Children requiring surgical intervention. His treatise involved an in-depth examination including huge laboratory and X-ray studies, with key histories and physicals of parent's, grandparent's and sibling's on each side of the family. This surgeon had dealt with the surgical techniques for Spina Bifida and their prognosis the outcome of such surgery. This treatise took into account all the known physiological functions, laboratory results, age-related mentation, and neuronal growth expectations.

After meeting with the Ward staff, his second proposal was to discuss all aspects of Baby Anne's progress, essentially so he would not to miss any nuance of the Baby's activities. His proposal would be to explore the possibility of excising this sac of Cerebro Spinal Fluid-before the sac grew any larger. The history of this type of surgery was grim, but it might be the only chance for a long-term survival. The previous and historical statistics of this dramatic surgery showed only scant survival and was based on Spina Bifida sac's at half the size of Baby Anne's bulging sac. The surgery was in its technique relatively simple for reducing the sac's size, but once the sac was cut, it then required extreme dexterity in suturing. Next, getting the repaired spinal cord tissues to lie in place again in the bones of the spinal column is fraught with difficulties. Even when the sac, with the two forceps clamped in place at skin level allowing the scalpel to cut through the tissue between the two forceps, creates a massive neurogenic shock with the sudden change in the sac's Cerebro Spinal Fluid. This massive 'shock' to the brain with the sudden loss of CSF as well as the its vital pressure. Obviously this was extremely dangerous, the loss of circulation fluid was problem one; problem two was the circulating pressure changing instantly leading to problem three, massive shock.

Once the clamped sac closest to the spine was clamped it needed to be sutured closed, then with incredible skill pushed back inside the still open bones of the vertebral column, these bones having been pushed and kept open by the protruding sac. If this technique of inserting the spinal cord or simply its cord's membrane back into the spinal column was done, the next major task was keeping the newly repaired 'cord' inside the two 'open' vertebras that needed to be closed! These spinal bones, that give us strength to keep our body erect, had to be fused back together or held together by a metal bridge which would be screwed into the vertebrae above and below the previously opened protrusion. This procedure required the great expertise of both the Pediatric Neurosurgeon and the Pediatric Orthopedic Surgeon, and on a seven-month-old baby even the Anesthesiologist would need to be extremely careful for an inordinate lengthy operation. The prognosis after the operation was poor, dismal.

Part of this second proposal also required a truthful, delicate and careful family discussion with the parents of Baby Anne. The decision-making was open to all her family members and those that cared for this baby girl. The prognosis for this extraordinarily beautiful little baby girl with her cherubic features was becoming critical, even as she was alive. Her Spina Bifida was obviously growing and even without the tenuous, fragile surgery that would last for many hours, she might die with the Spina Bifida sooner rather than later. She could die from the myriad complications of the post surgical period, which would include, more than likely a deadly staphylococcal infection. The odds of a successful surgical intervention, even with the finest surgical minds operating and working in harmony together, were against her.

Doctor Varley would give the parents the final decision, and he would give them all the possible outcomes, all of the issues as sad as they were, all they would have to consider, nothing would be left out. *Nothing*!

Doctor Varley contacted the Harley Street Pediatric Neurosurgeon, who had written exhaustively on infant and child spinal surgeries and he had replied. The information our Pediatrician had already gathered could not be expounded upon or changed, it was just as Doctor Varley had thoroughly researched. There were only the remaining choices of which of the specialists from the regional hospital system he would be consulting, and would come to do the surgery.

Transferring Baby Anne to another hospital facility, much further away would be another probably better choice, even though that pediatric specialized surgical unit was really familiar with this kind of spinal surgery. The parents had already clearly emphasized they did not want any other facility to care for their Baby daughter, especially if it was even further away from their home than we were. They wanted no extra travel time than our hospital already presented; the travel had become real hardship for them and their other three children.

A Saturday was chosen for the family conference. Along came Dad and Mum, with their three children, four sets of grand parents and their Vicar; the man to whom they sought spiritual advice and comfort. We all met in Sister Sandra Desmondhalgh's office and besides Sister Sandra, Staff Nurse Jennifer Foxhouse and myself were there. We had to move a desk and file cabinet's out of the office to make room for all the chairs, it was a little cramped but this kept the discussion an intimate family affair.

From the beginning, it seemed as though these loving and caring parents of Baby Anne sensed the gravity of this sad decision making time. From the birth of Baby Anne they knew the critical short time their child might have to be a part of their family, and up to this seventh month of Baby Anne's life she had always been hospitalized, so it was already a physical separation that had been endured. For two months I had been a major part of this child's life and I was heartbroken for them, realizing this conference was a life making or taking decision!

Doctor Varley, in his gentlest of voices, kindest tone and most loving fatherly manner, (for he too was a father of two boys), began by going over the events that may have occurred during pregnancy, and all suppositions. He made it very clear there was absolutely nothing the mother could have done to prevent having a baby with Spina Bifida. It was simply and completely an unknown factor, an anomaly and it occurred in every population in every country. He wanted to be certain that neither parent in their imagination or through their emotions would feel any guilt.

He explained that he had sought help and suggestions from the top Harley Street Surgical Specialist and University minds, in seeking out a successful outcome for this baby girl of theirs. He explained what would happen to this sac in exacting detail during the surgery and how it would affect Baby Anne including what demands on her tiny body it would require. Doctor Varley wanted the parents and any of the family to ask questions, allowing time to let their hearts and minds search for an understanding and come to an eventual decision. He told them that they did not need to make the decision right now since this day was set up for the conference and to all the relative information they needed to make this incredibly sad and so difficult decision. Doctor Varley asked them to let him know their wishes by the following Saturday when they came back for their weekly visit.

To all their questions, the chances of survival for this child of *unimagined beauty* were very slim at best, when the conference ended, there were essentially three choices for them. First, do surgery and pray for God's hand on the surgeons skill; second, to continue with Baby Anne to be in our care until her life ended with the sac erupting due to its increasing size; or third, take Baby Anne home with them and allow the same course of events-as leaving her in hospital with us.

Obviously, the only rare hope for her survival was to do surgery, but they clearly understood that the chances were not good and Baby Anne would have a long and perhaps torturous recovery. *With heavy hearts, after spending the next three hours at their child's cot and holding her and feeding her the applesauce she seemed to enjoy, they finally left with tears streaming down all their faces.* It was so sad, the adults crying and heads bowed low, the three siblings not totally comprehending the events but knowing this was frightening to their parents, they cried too and held each others hands. All the grandparents and the Vicar followed behind them arm-in-arm. Their vicar, a pleasant and kindly older man could only help them grieve and shared his tears with theirs.

Once outside the Peds Ward, on the walkway, the Vicar stopped and apparently asked everyone to hold hands and make a small circle. Everyone bowed their heads as they prayed for God to intervene for Baby Anne, for the child's recovery and for her to feel no pain or discomfort as the Spina Bifida grew and perhaps ruptured. As the Vicar prayed for the family also to be in God's grace with peace amongst this present suffering I went from standing outside the Ward's doorway saying my own private 'goodbyes', and joined the circle.

After they had all left, the Sisters office back to normal, I too left and I remember tears splashing over my checks. *A gift of a Baby Girl with such unimagined beauty, with such a perfect peace about her being given what seemed to be only a momentary life!* Remarkably, perhaps, I still remember so clearly all these years later-her angelic face and the peace that surrounded her! Indeed it did seem like her life was going to end soon, Doctor Varley had intimated quietly to me that Baby Anne's Spina Bifida had already extended beyond what is normally seem at our baby's age, and not be to surprised if the sac burst or collapsed even momentarily.

That night, going to bed, there was no joy in my heart. I cried for Baby Anne, her parents, her whole family *and I cried for myself.* Five days later, in the dark, quiet night hours two days before the parents had to make a decision, Baby Anne died in her sleep. Her bulging sac of Cerebro-Spinal fluid could not contain the pressure, and *ruptured ending her life.* Quietly, instantly.

I came on to the Pediatric Ward that Thursday morning and from the Ward entrance, I saw that her cot had been moved; instinctively I knew she was gone. Shorty after she had been admitted into my care I had taken a photograph of my Baby Anne whilst she was propped up on pillows in her cot and there, almost sitting, she was beaming at me with such a glorious angelic smile, at that moment heaven must have smiled too. I captured that unimagined beauty in a photo, and there she lives, in my album, in my memory!

For the next four or five days my heart was heavy, I was sad for me. This angelic baby had died peacefully in her sleep, I hoped, and it was probably for the best for the child herself and for the family. If she had gone through the torturous surgery and then died or had major complications, perhaps the loss of use of her legs, ability to control her bladder or her bowel movements. The most probably complication would be a massive and destructive infection that would not respond to the intravenous antibiotics. This would have created a dreadful and most difficult problem to resolve, an infection could have creep up into her brain, via the surgical site of the exercised Spina Bifida. Likewise the life-taking infection could insidiously destroy the blood stream affecting every organ of her body and like a treacherous enemy attacking every organ and life itself.

Baby Anne, as this lovely child who knew nothing of her plight, not even seeing the bulging mass on her back, nor even complaining, or only crying occasionally when hunger or a wet nappy disturbed her. She was a perfect little patient and I loved her as such. I could have loved her as my daughter and I think everyone else on the Pediatric Ward loved this baby. If love could have cured her, and there was so much love, she would have grown to become a radiant, beautiful, healthy woman, *for she was loved.*

Since this happened in my third year, and my Nursing skills were growing, I had become a good listener and seemed to be more attentive to things previously missed by my eyes, now these observation skills together with a greater ability to listen to the sounds of a re-bounding belly from a hand placed gently over the skin and the action of a bent finger tip hitting the other hands' outstretched finger so that the sound of this palpation returned a solid 'thud' or a hollow echo, I was feeling generally pleased with myself.

In learning, I was always a slow reader, but quite a respectable artist, and so, in anatomy and physiology, I drew bones, skin structures, nerve complexes, and a variety of microscopic invading bugs, from cocci, bacilli and viruses. Where I was slow in reading, often having to re-read passages, I seemed to be really good in memorizing anatomy and physiology, which after all was the foundation upon which everything else rested.

I remember reading with great interest how Michael Angelo Buonarroti, this Florentine sculptor, painter and architect had studied corpses and skeletons in the city morgue late in the evening hours to help him fully understand how human anatomy connected. He understood muscles working with other muscles how and where they attached to bone structures, with tissues beneath the skin, and blood vessels miraculously cobwebbed our body. He understood the complex mechanics of our body. This truly remarkable renaissance master of the fifteenth century, even in his simple drawings could clearly show a limb rotating to its fullest extent. Not me however, I painstakingly drew and corrected until the positions was right.

So, perhaps with a romanticized notion of learning how better to draw a bone or skull or even to get a better in-depth perspective view of how the skin peeled back showing muscles to be dissected and even on to the deeper bony prominences, I was ready, in this third year of mine to watch and even take part in a Post Mortem in our hospital morgue.

I still had another month to go to finish the Pediatric Rotation, but the opportunity arose for those third year nursing students who wanted to join the Pathologist, our American, Phil Ericson III for three days with him in the morgue. He kindly expressed the experience as, 'research post mortems'. Sounded good to eager Student Nurses.

I was excited, I could take my drawing pad and pencils, perhaps even my battered old camera that still worked, so that I too could get a 'renaissance man' vision of first hand anatomy. After asking the Nursing Tutor, David Howarth, if I could join him and the Pathologist he agreed and appreciated my enthusiasm. My excitement mounted for the Wednesday, Thursday and Friday to be in the Morgue, an artist observer or an assistant, I was ready for both.

My day off that week was Tuesday, before the Wednesday Morgue appointment. So I went to the local library and borrowed,

'The Life and Times of Michelangelo'. I studied lots of the superb illustrations, the simple line drawings to the complex intricate drawings of head and skull, of shoulders, chest and abdomen, of pelvis bone with muscle attachments to the legs. The femur, feet and delicate toes of small bodies, I wanted to be ready, after all, the Boy Scout motto of 'Be prepared' hung in my mind.

Wednesday arrived and I was early to get to this anticipated experience of sharpening nursing skills as well as it being an artistic exploration of form and absolute reality, no book illustrations here!

In the foyer of the Morgue, our Nursing Tutor David Haworth began with a brief overview of how very important post mortems were in both the actual determination of a death, and from a research point of view. He explained how 'medicine in general' would be better understood and hopefully where valuable insights would be learned and so shared with the medical community at large. Pathologist's findings had their own annals of scientific discovery.

Since there were only eleven Students Nurses attending, our Tutor and the Pathologist we were having this 'introduction' outside the Pathologist office, which was the foyer-almost a room in itself away from the Morgue, the light in this darkened basement area seemed to add to the air of a medical mystery. Our Tutor, after this very brief introduction, reintroduced Doctor Phil Ericson III, our Pathologist speaking his best American, who was anxious to begin since there were several post mortems to perform. He briefly related some stories of post mortems beginning in his early Cook Country General Hospital career in Chicago where, on one occasion, had to put back together, mainly for identification, four young men who were travelling very fast in a Volkswagen Beetle which hit a concrete post at the side of a main road severing heads and limbs from bodies, and torso's badly mutilated on their super high speed collision, completely ripping the Volkswagen into two mangled sections. A horrific scene, creating a non-stop four-day autopsy jigsaw, arduous work for all the Pathologists and their students!

Doctor Ericson's last post mortem, done here on Monday; two days earlier had been on a young woman from the Surgical Ward. This poor lady's diagnosis had been Colon and Rectal Carcinoma, and after the enormously long and complex surgery, the 'Abdominal Peritoneal Resection' where two surgeons worked at the same time, one going into the abdomen, and the second excising away through the Perineal area. This surgery required the second surgeon to sit below the elevated operating table and perform the surgery between the patient's legs, which were held high on the table's stirrups. The surgery had been done three weeks earlier. Her post operative recovery was fraught with massive amounts of pain, inability to move her legs, a Colostomy that was first inactive, then simply continued to bleed and crowned over everything was her hyper-pyrexial fever that even the full strength intravenous antibiotics had no effect upon. The surgeon, on the provisional Death Certificate had written *'Septicaemia Secondary to Surgery for Colonic-Rectal Cancer'*. Doctor Ericson's post mortem conclusion verified the surgeons finding but added *'Gross Carcinogen Invasion of the entire Abdominal and Pubic Cavity'*. A sad outcome for a surgery that lasted six and a half hours! Pathology was not the happiest of subjects he said, but like finding that Tetanus Spore, dropping from the decaying plaster of the operating rooms' ceiling, the Epidemiology and Pathology discovery had its moment of victory and glory.

From the Foyer he ushered us all into the Morgue that was dimly lit, but the light above the morgue table was similar to the powerful light in the operating room. There were four huge refrigerators for the four bodies that were presently residing there, however only two of the bodies were there for Doctor Ericson's post mortem investigation. He had his morgue orderly open each fridge to show us the sheet covered bodies and the inside of the fridge's.

Then, on a meticulously arranged large surgical tray that articulated over his morgue table, this table he to it referred as *'the slab'*, the articulating tray contained similar looking surgical instruments to the operating room but with added saws of different designs to saw through thick or thin bones. There was an electrical saw and a drill. He called the orderly to bring his first body, the white sheet being removed as he brought the body and laid it on the cold metal slab.

It was my Baby Anne. The Pediatrician and the parents wanted to know what anomaly had possibly caused the Spina Bifida; much more 'research' was necessary to find a cause, which would lead to a possible cure, they had been told, so of course they agreed to the post mortem—*on this tiny body!*

Now this child's body, lifeless and cold, the flushed gentle pink of her cheeks now turned a pale, waxen unkind gray colour, this tiny child looked even smaller than in life. I shivered in anxiety, feeling tears begin to roll down my cheeks as the morgue orderly placed a u-shaped wooden support under Anne's limp head. Her head wobbled from side to side when he did this and as I looked into this angelic face again, tears flowed freely cascading over my cheeks. I felt a supporting, tender hand of one of my nurse colleagues' as she squeezed my hand knowing that Baby Anne had been under my care.

Doctor Ericson, a scalpel in hand, made one long incision around my baby's head. I gasped tearfully out loud, a frantic cry for all babies with Spina Bifida! Running blindly, I stumbled out of the morgue, never going back to see another post mortem. Nor will I ever again.

The days of Michaelangelo and his nightly adventures to draw, dissect, compare or discover the human anatomy and its mechanics were over.

His illustrations of cold, dead bodies where no love was involved could now safely stay in books on the shelf, away from my eyes and very recent memory. And the cause of the anomaly for my Baby Patient, the reason for my Baby Anne's death was never resolved.

* I no longer remember the last name of Baby Anne's parents, but should they ever read my book, and remember their Baby in our care at the hospital on the hill, of a great Pediatrician and those superb Nurses that loved their daughter-I had taken a photo of her, smiling peacefully, beautifully I would be honoured to give them that photo!

CHAPTER 10

INVALID COOKERY

Bedpans for Breakfast and Kidney Dishes for Lunch-Shakespearian Style

Being a First year Student Nurse was actually quite hard work, frequently getting onto whichever Ward one was assigned by seven am and, depending on the day or the rotation, it meant cleaning, and more cleaning. Wooden floorboards of the Ward needed cleaning, so moving all the beds from one side of the Ward to the other, sweeping then polishing those boards and repeating the process for the opposite side. Then, wet or dry dusting cleaning of the Ward furniture, then on to the more glorious cleaning tasks of scrubbing bedpans, urinals, kidney-dishes, syringing through the red rubber tubing used for intravenous blood transfusions or IV medications, then popping them into the huge sterilizers. Glorious cleaning. However, there was a time during period this First year that we got to enjoy a respite of two weeks during that year where we escaped the Fortress Hospital to learn all about Invalid Cookery at an older TB Hospital. This sounded like we should be able to cook all kinds of 'invalid' foods and devour them on the spot all hot and steamy fresh, and we would get to eat them for free. How gourmet can we become, Invalid Cookery indeed. Well, the main reason of course was to teach us Nutrition, about food groups and where

180

starch's, proteins, vitamins come from. We were to learn how carbohydrates, sugars and all foods eventually become energy. Where our digestive process creates our B.M.R., the Basic Metabolic Rate, this fascinating measurement where we establish a rate where a body is at complete rest, and measure energy used at this very basic level of life. Information that will stay with us for the rest of our lives, this knowledge of our body generating heat in a 'unit of time' is recognized as calories used per kilogram of body weight. Calories, metabolic rates, energy expended, so basically we are going to really enjoy this change in all of our B.M.R's as we leave the cleaning, sweeping and polishing of our Wards for the gentle Classroom cum Kitchen for two weeks of creative, *cooking and consuming* our own gourmet dishes. Who can beat this?

In gentle command of this Invalid Cookery School for Nurses was the sweetest of Nursing Sister's. Her name was Sister Beryl Spencer, and I would guess her age at sixty although she could have been older. Instead of the dark navy blue dress, which almost all sisters wore, no matter which hospital you were in throughout Britain, Sister Spencer wore a forest green dress and it gave her a more noble, perhaps a more royal appearance. Her lovely high white and thoroughly starched cap was crowned with a beautiful Nottingham Lace around its top edges. Her forest green dress was belted at her waist with an ample darker green band for a belt, with a Buckle upon which had a Coat of Arms badge attached to it. The buckle, she later told us was a memorial for, *"The finest woman that ever lived. This is my Florence Nightingale memorial belt buckle".* Indeed, she wore it with pride. The cuffs on her sleeves were trimmed with the same exquisite lace as her cap giving her a commanding appearance.

Her dress reached below her knees, showing nicely shaped legs clad in heavy black cotton stockings, and a final touch of class was evident in the Italian leather shoes of a dark green colour-indeed, which was unusual too. The darker green belt around her waist, with its Buckle harmonized with her shoes that were also adorned with sparkling, square silver buckles. We instantly loved this more mature and quite unique Lady Nurse. Her age did not affect the elegance of this lady of the *'buckles'*, buckle on waist and buckles on her shoes. But this was just the beginning.

Her welcoming for us from our hospital, (many hospital's within the fairly large hospital region) sent their first year Student Nurses here, in a rotation that kept her invalid cookery class going almost all year, so her 'welcomes' to each class was probably quite routine. This first introduction from her seemed like we were her first class she had ever taught. She made us feel important, even valuable! She beamed a glorious smile that lit her gently furrowed brown, this lovely smile seemed like a permanently sculpted fixture to her gentle face but it was a genuine smile. Her lips opened showing perfectly straight white teeth, and her oval shaped face was emblazoned with silvery grey hair, tresses of hair hiding her ears, but what a smile, and this was our welcome.

Sister Spencer introduced herself, giving us a brief history of her adventures across the world of so long ago in China first, then as a missionary and later spending many years in North Africa, the Sudan and Egypt. She became a nurse later in life, actually her late thirties, this itself was unusual, since the vast majority of Student Nurses entered into nursing before reaching twenty years old. This Lady was a life-experienced woman that had already accomplished much long before she had began Nurses Training. It was she, that after qualifying as an SRN and then began working in a Tuberculosis Sanitarium who had convinced the Administrative Hospital Council that Nurses, whilst going through their first year of classes, should be taught the vital importance of Nutrition and how frail patients needed special, easily digestible foods to regain their health more rapidly. The Hospital Council had apparently believed too, and that if their long-term stay patients could be given nutritious foods it would decrease their hospitalization, hence saving health care expenses, a brilliant proposition.

This was how this pioneering, mature lady nurse had been assigned the responsibility for teaching 'Invalid Cookery' in the older unused TB Wards that were turned into Cookery Classrooms, so here I was, ready to learn a new very usable skill.

The classroom Kitchen consisted of two fairly large rooms with several smaller rooms for offices, storage and supplies, it had been part of this much larger Tuberculosis and Tropical Disease Rehabilitation Hospital, where Sister Spencer had first become a

Staff Nurse, then promoted to Sister before her newly created position of Director of Dietary and Invalid Cookery.

Four days a week Sister Spencer was joined by her assistant Audrey Herarda, who was also a Staff Nurse, and who also had Nursed in a hospital in Nairobi, Kenya where her husband was, it seemed, a multi functioning Physician, doing surgery, tropical disease medicine, pathology and occasionally standing in as the obstetrician routinely delivering babies. Prior to Kenya he had spent 5 years in Singapore as an Army Physician with the Royal Army Medical Corp.

Staff Nurse Audrey Herarda was a blond, blue-eyed beauty of thirty-four or thirty-five; the males in our class made it a goal to get her to give us her age. She had a flirtatious flip of her head that would send her golden hair bunched up into a large bun at the back of her head into a fascinating tremor and at the same time her eye brows would suddenly more up on her forehead as her eyes opened wide. Was this momentary physical expression gave a flirtatious suggestion or just a genuine act of surprise, another mystery to unravel along the way, and a goal to accomplish, this dietary stuff and its associated benefits were getting more exciting.

Staff Nurse Herarda was a beauty too, in both her facial features and her bodily attributes in her dark blue uniform dress, she too wore a wide tight belt, which exaggerated her waist and cut a perfect shape of a perfect woman! This, at least, was the learned opinion of all the Male Nurses that met her. Audrey's role was to be the roving teacher between all the separate, stoves, and ovens and cook tops, where each student had their own cooking area as well as all the pots and pans that were required. Each day was to be a new culinary adventure. The mornings were classroom orientation and the afternoons were the hands-on experience, sadly, not on Staff Nurse Audrey, but actually cooking. There were days when we had all finished early. We had prepared, cooked or baked or fried a variety of dishes then ate and 'tested' them, generally with much gusto. The morning formal classroom tuition under Sister Spencer was always interesting, colourful and filled with why different diseases required different nutritional approaches; alternatively with a gastric malady that might involve gall bladder, peptic ulcer or liver, or perhaps with the difficult progression of a Crohns Disease. There were diets, on diets and simple nutrient diets. Diets for ulcers, or obstructions in the lower end of the intestine, diets for the Mentally ill and diets for nursing Mothers. If there was not a 'diet' for a particular disease, she could have created one. All these medical problems needed slightly different approaches to digestion and our body's need of adequate nutrition and hydration. There was a time to eat and a time for NPO-nothing by mouth!

We learned it all; we became Master Chefs-our own assessment of our own skills! We made flavourful chicken broth, custards and jelly's with new tastes, we baked sweet breads with honey and a touch of treacle or ginger, and we dished eggs into all manner of boiled, poached and scrambled creations. This was invalid cookery heaven, was made even more memorable with the extended lunch periods. During our class day, we had our Lunch Break, but we knew we would be eating soon after the 'official' lunch. With this spare time period we learned how to become great actors and actresses during this break in our day.

The huge rehabilitation hospital spread over several acres had many buildings; and many Wards had been empty for long periods of time. These Wards were still filled with beds, sterilizers, wheel chairs, intravenous equipment, and trolleys for patients and wheeled carts for instruments, and there were even those massive, amazing iron lungs. Theses Wards became our Theatre, a homemade Opera House, a Grand Stage an idea of the Old Globe. Within a well filled, full of equipment Ward we collectively decided we could become 'more than we were', so we became for most of these break periods, comic Actors and Actresses or stars of the Stage and Opera! The linen rooms on these Wards still held counter-panes, draw sheets and regular sheets and pillowcases. It was from this lovely horde of linen we made gowns for the ladies and both short capes for musketeers or long flowing robes for Lords and Ladies of the Realm. Bedpans became our stainless steel helmets and kidney dishes doubled as shoulder and knee armour – kept in place by old, but still sticky, surgical tape.

We used infant prams or baby carriages for imaginary Horses in a Jousting Tournament, or a Stage Coach of the old West, on more daring escapades around the Ward or out to the interconnecting corridors we would use the longer stainless steel stretchers whose wheels creaked and moaned as they were put back into use after being stationary for many years. Intravenous poles, broom handles and even antiquated long sponge holding forceps became prop weapons for the *age of chivalry,* our play-acting. We were serfs from the village, or courtiers from a Princely Court of some mystical country land in the renaissance times of rebirth, revival and a renewed shinning human experience. We were the first of the Elizabethan actors of Shakespeare's 'Old Globe', as we recreated his comedies, tragedies and histories indeed we were the bard's players. On one occasion, we created our own operating room, we made all the furniture into sterilizers, anesthesia carts, and found a bright large floodlight, which we rigged into the overhead light position, and became our operating light under which we placed a stainless steel stretcher which was now the operating table. To make our operating room more 'realistic' we surrounded our operating room with the privacy screens that had wheels for easy mobility. And finally found two huge green sheets that would become the 'doors' to the operating room. And for the final touch of realism, as the doors on our hospitals operating room wrote on the sheets *'In, No Smoking'* and the other *'Out, No Smoking'*. This set-up had taken us two lunchtime break periods and it would be our final play, our Grand Finale. The Student Nurse team of nine, would all be involved playing a separate character from our own Operating Room staff, including our eccentric surgeons and anesthesiologist, whom we knew well. Now we needed a real life 'actress' patient, and we all decided the perfect person would be our Staff Nurse Audrey Herarda of our infamous Invalid Cookery class.

Our blond flirtatious beauty, who we thought may be a little uncomfortable with the role of patient, and since we wanted her hair out of the bun style back to freely flowing hair down to her shoulders, and we wanted her to wear our makeshift hospital gown a bit risky perhaps when we asked her to get up onto our operating table and ready for our imaginary surgery. But would she even agree to the part?

I took the responsibility to approach Audrey Herarda and ask her to do something she may never have thought about doing before. At the end of our second week, at the end of our lesson I stayed back and perhaps somewhat timidly approached her with the basic idea of our break time drama to be put on at the end of our course and after the final exam. It would be a Grand Finale Salute, a kind of 'Thank You' effort to Sister Spencer, a gesture Audrey may not be able to refuse. She neither agreed nor disagreed, but told me she would think about it and let me know the following Tuesday. That Tuesday arrived and I tenaciously approached her again. She told me she had visited the Ward in which we had created our 'old globe' operating room, and said she was generally amazed at our efforts in rediscovering a use for these 'props'. She kindly said that all those hospital items, after we had finished with them, should be packed up and sent to some hospital in Africa where they could be a real value! She would agree to do this 'skit' providing we would put pillows on the operating room table to make it comfortable for her and finally, this play acting had to be done on the last Friday of our schedule, and the other major agreement, besides inviting Sister Beryl Spencer, we had to invite all the other nurses from the TB Hospital who could get off for an hour-as our guests. Our regal and royal performance was going to be attended by many more than we had originally anticipated, but that was the price of stardom!

With a sliver of anxiety, thinking that Sister Spencer would perhaps be annoyed and ask us to get rid of our 'misuse of hospital property' and put everything back in its place, she graciously accepted saying that she was aware that her Invalid Cookery Students were up to some improbable or mischievous antics. From Tuesday to Thursday we nine Invalid Cookery Students rehearsed our parts. We were going to mimic our favourite Surgeon, and his Indian House Surgeon's Doctor's Rajeev Singh and Jitish Raza who had newly arrived at our hospital and spoke the English language with a lovely strong Indian accent from his home state of Manipur and his region of Kakching. He had shared this information with us on a recent late evening during his rounds. All of us could easily remember 'Kakching' and pronounced it with a lovely Peter Seller's cum Indian accent, however, Doctor Raza himself was very hard to understand and whenever he was giving us orders for a patient he had to write everything down for clarity. We referred to him in our best effort of English-Indian as Doctor Kakching and, sometimes it sounded like 'ka-ching', the sound of money going into in the till!

We would also impersonate the Anesthesiologist in his finest blustery anger and his red-faced fury; we made the Operating Room Sister and her Staff Nurse who frequently answered our questions sarcastically. We made the less liked Gynecologist have his tantrums and in fits of either frustration, anger or whatever, would throw an instrument from the Operating Room Table to the far corner of the room, oh, how dare he be so arrogant. We presented the O.R. orderly as a pure delight of a man who could tell the best of clean and 'off colour' jokes, for this performance they would be clean and really funny.

The last two parts would be first year nurses who were just learning how to put those oversized, very uncomfortable stainless steel bed pans into the a bed where a patient had to remain flat in bed, this always brought peals of laughter as the nurse struggled endlessly to get it right as the patient complained venomously about having their bottoms cut to pieces by this metal monstrosity, and the total lack of privacy, no dignity.

We were finally ready, our Invalid Cookery creations tasted, tried and enjoyed, the nutrient values learned and recorded, the final exam of sorts a cooked dish of steamed fish and an essay of why we thought this special class was of particular importance.

Now all of that was behind us, we were cooks of repute! Now it was time to become the actors and actresses for our final performance, and it must be good. Our reputations would perhaps hang on this event till the end of our Student Nursing days. Glorious thought. Everyone went over to the disused Ward where we had created our grand stage of Elizabethan promise.

The operating room door, the No Smoking door, opened into our operating room of three sides, the forth side we had placed one bed and several chairs to be used for the other staff. Sister Beryl was our V.I.P. so she would sit on the bed, this was her own 'balcony' to appreciate our drama, and hopefully cheer us on.

The primary excitement for the four male student actors, myself as their leader was in the preparation of Staff Nurse Audrey. This was our pre-performance highlight. She arrived, after going home earlier, so she could change out of her uniform, and now her blonde hair surrounded a lovely face that could have been used in a Hair Shampoo advertisement.

She looked spectacular. However, and disappointingly, we had expected a tight pullover cardigan or even buttoned blouse and a shorter skirt than her nursing uniform, but in dismay we saw she was wearing a loose fitting full-length dress that had a polo-neck design. So, we were not going to see much bare skin, upon which to perform our surgery, so we had to enjoy her hair and face. She may have suspected that we wanted to appreciate all her lovely attributes-during our play-as well as more skin, but she was smarter than we! She had understood our determined stares at her dress, and what we may have been expecting, planning and hoping, artistically speaking of course!

We got our patient on the operating room table, made her as comfortable as we could and it was then that a terrible thought crossed my mind, I should not have been playing the role of Doctor David Peter Alexander our incredibly gifted yet utterly eccentric surgeon, I should have been that frightfully angry, never ever happy, our senior Anesthesiologist Doctor Dennis Holt! I had miscalculated for it would be this frequently red faced man, giving the patient anesthesia that would be at the head of our operating room table and hence play the part of lurching over our patient-Staff Nurse Audrey Herarda. Her head and face would also be relatively close to him as he '*pretended*' to deliver anesthesia. Oh too late, I would only be able to approach the operating table and pull off the green O.R. towels that would be covering the imaginary abdominal operating site. Well, I would have to make do with the secret glances that I could make to look upon her face-hopefully-with her eyes closed under our pretended anesthesia period. I could, if brave enough, put a little extra pressure on her abdomen as a removed the green towels with the intent of pulling out of the wound a length of intestine! All the lads in this half hour play probably had similar imaginings of how they would gently touch our blond model of a patient.

Between us, we had talked about it. How about frequently checking her blood pressure, we could make sure the arm cuff was as high up on her arm as possible, but these little masculine testosterone driven ideations disappeared as the female student nurse actresses did these more delicate tasks; another brilliant idea gone to the sterile bucket.

The play began, we all played our parts, our lovely patient was enthusiastic and understanding, our audience giggled and laughed out loud as we mimicked in words and actions to our best with our Indian intonations of the English language recreated from our Senior Surgical Residents.

After our well deserved applause, and after we had finally put everything back in its place it was time for our parting. Our good-byes were memorable for the three weeks we had been on this wonderful interlude that everyone had enjoyed. The gentle, warm and affirming attention of Sister Beryl Spencer and her colleague Staff Nurse Audrey Herarda, were both bright shining lights for us. We had thoroughly appreciated all the 'invalid foods' we had prepared, cooked and eaten, but especially our lunch break times had actually been fun. Our acting antics, and the mimicking of our hospital physicians in an instantly created stage setting in that disused Hospital Ward was the proverbial icing on our invalid cooking cake.

So now, to return to the daily cooking sterilizers and those unending requests for bed pans, kidney dishes and a range of miasma-like unpleasant smells!

Oh where is that compote of custard?

CHAPTER 11

The Mental Ward

Glorious Psychiatry 'For Whom the Key's Roll', Dreams of Scottish Glens

Perhaps by simple coincidence, rather than a cleverly devised plot by the dark forces of the Fortress complex, the Mental Hospital of one hundred and sixty beds was the gloomiest, and it was located in the center of all the other buildings, perhaps they were guarding it. To me it was the most dismal, darkest gray building of all the different Wards, departments and outlaying hospital divisions that the Fortress Hospital possessed.

Its walls around its complete circumference were higher than any other building. The windows were widely spaced; narrower and erected higher up the wall from the interior floor-actually needing a stepladder to reach the interior windowsill. The roof of this eagerly named Mental Hospital had the steepest, most difficult roof to ever think of a *'great escape'*. The roof, like all the buildings built at the same time, was tiled with black slate and the maintenance crew would probably resign their jobs rather than go up on this roof to replace a broken or dislodged slate tile.

There were no gardens around any part of this ominous looking building; however it did have a tall, three-foot wide Privet Shrub around most of its walls. This was either a brilliant idea or a gardeners answer to Safety First; certainly it would have helped to break any fall of some adventurous patient trying to escape any of the darkened Ward's of the Mental Hospital from any window to the hopeful light of day. Alternatively, had some maintenance fellow ventured up on to the dangerously sloping roof to repair a tile and lost his footing, and falling to the ground below, had the distinct possibility of landing on the Privet bushes. That person would escape death, enduring only slight cuts and skin tears from the branches rather than a solid 'whack' that would probably leave him lifeless! So the gardeners cared for these perennial plants by trimming them carefully, but perhaps not realizing their future benefit as lifesavers.

The front entrance was the only interruption to the smooth walls around the rest of this building. The architect, in all of his creative skills and maybe a sense of humour or perhaps an incredible understanding of urban planning cost analysis had at the end of the only a one car narrow driveway, had three steps from the building that squarely came out to meet the short driveway. After these three steps another short landing of about six feet then a second series of three steps, each step shorter than the last up to the heavy wooden door, upon which was hung a large brass doorknocker. These steps brought patients and visitors alike, up to the front door. Incidentally, the huge heavy doorknocker required someone with exercised muscles to pull it and knock! Otherwise, you may have to wait a moment or two, or three.

Once inside this edifice of learning and reflection, the light from outside disappeared immediately the huge front door closed of its own accord. If you were an architectural student the maze you found inside would make your head spin, a design with no design. However, if you were a patient and needed medication you would never know where you are at any one time, and this was frequently the problem for Visitors as well as Student Nurses coming in for their Psychiatric Rotation. But we were ready for *any confusion of any kind.*

There were five Wards of twenty beds each for males and four Wards of fifteen beds for females. The corridors beyond the admitting area at the front of the hospital had both long and short corridors, these corridors sometimes intersected where the longer corridors ended with a Ward at its end. The corridors were tiled in the usual 'hospital green' colour and were noisy if anyone wore leather shoes. Every corridor had a locked door at both its beginning an end. This was a building for a Locksmiths delight.

The kitchen where all the meals were prepared was at the rear of the building, and it was through the kitchen door to the outside, where supplies came in for both the meals and the dry goods, toilet paper, office supplies and so on. The back door, cleverly hidden from view by the design of the wall that surrounded the whole building, had to be manually opened with a person holding the door. Once open, beyond the door it led on to a high walled courtyard where delivery trucks had tight access, one truck at a time, and they had to come through a massive double gate with heavy latches and locks both inside and out, which if opened had to be physically held open until a delivery was made.

Where the meal carts and trolleys came out of the kitchen into the large dining room, there was a stairway that led up into the upper treatment rooms, a series of four rooms approximately twenty by twenty feet. One room held supplies of dressings, drugs, linens and dry supplies, another room held a variety of equipment, patient tables, examining tables, stools, cabinets on wheels and the patient bed screens with their wheels. The other two rooms were kindly, if anything, called *'Treatment Rooms.'* These were the days of Electric Shock Therapy where electrodes were placed on each side of the head; to the front of the ears and varying electrical currents of power would zap through the frontal lobe of the brain! A wooden tongue depressor, an airway of sorts, would be put in the patients mouth just prior to the shock so that the unfortunate patient did not bite off a piece of his or her tongue. These two rooms had identical equipment in them of patient tables, patient soft and solid leather restrains, medicine carts with their intravenous medications, anesthesia carts holding oxygen and nitrous oxide cylinders, a variety of black rubber airways and wooden tongue depressors, as well as syringes, bottles of intravenous solutions and tubing. There were always several vials of this wonderful drug, Coramine, the cardiac muscle stimulant with the twenty cc.

syringes and spinal needles, just in case we needed to do emergent and hopeful resuscitation with the *Needle in the Heart* routine!

For this Mental Hospital of both male and female patients we had two Nursing Sisters, a male and a female. For the male patients it was a male 'Sister' who was a gentle giant of an Irishman, an intelligent, bright, a philosopher of sorts with a great sense of humour. The Nursing Offices for the two 'Sisters' were separated on either side of the main corridor behind the admitting areas at the front of the hospital. Each Ward Sister had a Staff Nurse for each of their Wards with two orderlies on each Ward; all of the Staff Nurses and their orderlies for each Ward were all male nurses, and Female Wards with their staff equally all female staff. If help was needed on one side or the other, then it came from the opposite side. The Student Nurses, male and female were assigned during their three-month rotation on the appropriate Ward.

This is where I met Sister Mr. Larry Winifreds our gentle Irish philosopher, our male 'Sister' and the person who always did the welcoming speech for the newly rotating Student Nurses. He was a humourist and a historian, his speeches covered the realm of Mental Health and Psychiatric Nursing from the less glorious days of 'Bedlam', that infamous institution-more kindly, but less well known as the *'Hospital of Saint Mary of Bethlehem'*, in the City of London. It was the Lunatic Asylum or Mad House whose noisy confusion and wild uproars could be heard well beyond its cloistered walls. Beginning with its creation in the fourteenth century, *Bedlam's Wards and corridors were a constant pandemonium.* Its walls sometimes ready to burst with overcrowding; there was anguish, chaos and confusion at every turn. Both the poor Nursing Staff dealing with patients suffering from a variety of severe mental illness as well as the Physicians who hopefully were well educated enough in mental health, all trying to bring a modicum of sanctity to their patients. Even bringing a calm to the patient's relatives who for the most part believed that once a person crosses the threshold of Bedlams' door they would never see the light of day again. It was not a therapeutic place for anyone with a mild type of mental illness, and certainly not for anyone with a simple 'emotional issue'. No, this institution was created for those who were mad. Judges,

Policemen, Barristers and Lawyers of every kind sent these poor mentally insane creatures there. Their own families who could no longer cope with their noisy, selfish and destructive behavior occasionally brought them to Bedlam. It was possible too, that patients were brought to this mental lunatic asylum by scheming relatives who wanted them 'out of-the-way! And *thereby hangs a Dickens classic novel perhaps.*

Mr. Winifreds introduction to Psychiatric Nursing, besides covering the world of London's fabled Bedlam, covered the advances in the physical hospital setting, the latest scientific journeys into therapies of Electrical Shock Treatment, massive doses of drugs to treat exotic states of Catatonic rigidity or extreme flexibility of each limb whilst appearing to be in a major stupor. He discussed how, now in this enlightened time period of Medicine his own Psychiatric Ward would accept from the local police stations' prison, men and women who were incredibly drunk! These sad souls who were major Chronic Alcoholics, who coming into our Ward still vomiting up whatever might be left in their gastro-intestinal tract, but foolishly pleading for another drink. Mr. Winifreds told us of the classic treatment ordered by our Consultant Psychiatrist; Doctor John Ronald Andrews was first to get them to calm down then to begin the pathway back to sobriety. To do this we needed that ever ready, dreadful smelling Drug the injection of Paraldehyde. Inebriated or drunk, sometimes it took a whooping twenty cc's in each buttock, which caused cries of pain and burning! Yes, that was a huge amount of injectable fluid for anyone 40cc's in all, and the Paraldehyde was a viscous type of a solution that did not rapidly disperse into the surrounding tissues and blood supply. The smell of Paraldehyde that permeated the alcoholics Recovery Ward, the *'Tanked'* or *'Snockered' Ward*, as Mr. Winifreds smilingly called it. That odorous smell from the alcoholic's breath was due to the way in which the metabolic system processed the drug coming into the body. Utilizing this drug via the blood stream it would be partially excreted through the lungs, so that the patients breath stank of this foul odiferous drug. Paraldehyde has both been generally used as a hypnotic drug-a restful sleeping agent, and in our case, as an anti-convulsant drug as well as a hypnotic.

Mr. Winifreds discussed the role of psychiatrists, psychologists, and mental health workers and finally Mental Nurses-who had taken further study and exams after their SRN, General Nurses training. This topic of the 'pecking order of roles', from the mighty Psychiatrist to the lower social order of Psychologists, (according to Doctor Andrews that is), then to the 'rest of us', he really enjoyed, he actually relished this subject. "Everything", he declared, "depended on whether you were... *'to the manor born'*".

This further explanation made it clear that only the Psychiatrists have their Medical Degrees, as when Physicians become Psychiatrists, therefore the MD's! The Psychologists, on that lower rung of authority, had only PH.D degree, so in theory they had less knowledge than the MD, Psychiatrists. So, Mr. Winifreds put himself on an even lower rank, but for me, with his sound common sense he certainly was on an even higher rung than the chief! In the manor born, my Derriere! He knew his stuff, he *was* the man.

This lovely introduction was leading up to the list of characters that ruled his glorious Psychiatric Ward of ours. Here we were to learn of the great man *'for whom the keys roll'*!

As odd as this may seem, all the interior Psychiatric door keys, all forty-eight of them were kept in two round colourful Christmas biscuit tins! Each round biscuit tin held twenty-four keys for the Male Mental Wards, and twenty-four keys for the Female side of the Mental hospital. The biscuit tins were round and so could be rolled across a table, or whatever other flat surface, these tins had originally held biscuits to be sold at Christmas, for the colourful round side and top were illustrated with Christmas trees, churches, carolers and snowmen. On top of the tins were our own created labels, one with a letter 'M' the other with a letter 'F' for male or female Wards. The tins and their keys was the 'brain child' of our Psychiatrist-*'if the keys were in Biscuit Tins, no one would know the tins were full of keys'*! Oh well! The tins had to be kept in each Sisters office and they had to be up on the shelf above their desks and between old medical books of Psychiatric theory and practice, and with long out of date British Medical Journals.

The idea, I learned, was to keep the whole set of keys hidden from prying eyes. The tins had no camouflage but were brightly coloured; perhaps our August psychiatrist considered 'colour' as camouflage! The only time the keys were to be taken from these biscuit tins was when the great man himself would come to do his Ward Grand Rounds and he hung on to those keys as though he was the Warden of the Crown Jewels. I met this leading Consultant Psychiatrist on my first day on the Psychiatric Ward, after Sister Mr. Larry Winifreds descriptive overtures of both Doctor Andrews's personality and his demands of the staff for prompt attention to his every order. Our Doctor always arrived with exceedingly prompt perfection at exactly eleven am on the dot.

This dear fellow was the incredibly bizarre Psychiatrist and Senior Regional Mental Health Consultant, this indeed was Doctor John Ronald Andrews, and he may well have been off his rocker. Alas, who is to judge? His 6'4" height just allowed him to walk under the doors frame without bobbing his head down. His brown graying hair was parted exactly in the middle of his head, and he obviously used major grease that kept his hair glued to his scalp. His long thin face with pronounced ears sticking out like antennae had deep set eyes, straight yet powerful nose and a surprisingly small mouth and tight lips with an almost pointy chin. He was a serious man and may have forgotten how to smile, but he did have a commanding voice that did portray his belief that he was firmly in command of his world, and the world of this, his Mental Hospital. He was a meticulous dresser always attired in a grey or black suit and was one of the few physicians who wore a bow tie rather than the more usual ties. His bow ties were colourful and he changed them every day he came to do his rounds. I heard from Sister Mr. Larry that he probably had one bow tie for every patient he had on his roster.

During his Grand Rounds he clung on to the bunch of twenty-four keys. Each time he came into the hospital and popped into the Sister office, he would reach up to the shelf where his biscuit tin held those keys.

The patient's charts were all put into their separate hangers in the chart trolley, and once Doctor Andrews surveyed his grand entourage of Resident Psychiatric Physician, the Psychologist, Mental Health worker, Recreational Therapist, Sister Mr. Winifreds staff and Student Nurses. Once he approved of his rounding group would head to the first corridor door and he alone was the one who both unlocked the door and after everybody had passed through the door – passing him by, then he would turn back to lock the door. Each locking or unlocking of the doors he would nervously begin rolling those noisy keys from hand to hand. He did this with every door in the hospital and where ever the corridors led to patient Wards or examining rooms, he was 'rolling those keys' for someone, but who?

At the foot of every bed, and once the group had arrived and stood around the bed with him, he would ask the patient, if they were awake, a series of questions that he asked of every single patient either male or female. His questions in strict order were; 1. Do you know who I am? 2. Do you know why you are here? 3. Do you understand your illness or diagnosis? 4. Do you remember where you live? 5. What was the name of the last book you read? Some patients who were actually more mentally awake would jokingly reply 'Goldilocks' or 'Jack and the Beanstalk' then smile at our grand master who would righteously ignore their reply and smile. Almost everyone knew the answer to the first question and they either ignored or whispered "yes"; perhaps some fearing retribution if they said "no" then he would repeat the question and ask, 'so what is my name? If they simply replied, *"Doctor Andrews"*, he would correct them explaining his full name and title, *I'm Doctor John Ronald Andrews and I am your Consultant Psychiatrist!* He said this with pride and in a slightly higher tone of voice than before.

To the other questions, except 'do you know where you live?' there was always an immediate silence or a low murmured "No" or 'not sure' or 'can't remember". Apparently these memory questions served Doctor Andrews as a guide to their mental well-being or their deterioration. If there was no response to any questions, and the patient held their head down, not wanting to be confronted by so many people, or to see this mighty Doctor Andrews and all the staff surrounding his bed or simply that the patient was lost in a revere of days of long ago, and those memories were more peaceful than the drama of this present daily circus. To these unfortunate patients Doctor Andrews gave a seven day grace period to say something, anything, and if nothing at the end of this seven day *'mystical therapy'* of his, the patient would be further destined for electrical shock treatment to wake up whatever was not working in those frontal, or other lobes of his patients. It seemed to me, that this barbaric electrical shock of the poor old brain was used for everything, for 'manic' behavior, for severe anxiety, or severe depression and a variety of psychoses and other mental anomalies, or whenever Doctor Andrews seemed it to be in the patients 'best interest'.

This use of electroshock therapy was simple in its concept, send a powerful shock through the brain and hopeful it will disrupt, even change the present activity in the brain to bring about a healing or at least a change of behavior for the better we hoped. This Electro-Convulsive Therapy seemed to me like a *spark in the dark* at best, and having watched it, and followed up with the results, I never saw any improvement in any patients! Several times whilst doing my psych rotation in both my second and third year training, my part in all of this was to keep the tongue depressor-airway in the patient's mouth immediately after he was given the intravenous Sodium Pentothal that induced rapid unconsciousness. Once the tongue depressor–airway was in place, the electrodes were placed at the temples on each side of the head, then the Psychiatrist delivered the shock.

The electrical shock itself could actually cause unconsciousness, and a series of brief seizures, these convulsions ranged from mild–where only the head and shoulders would move erratically, to more sever convulsions where the whole body would violently contort. The strong leather restraining straps holding the patient down prevented the contortions from sending the patient flying. On each of my brief sojourns on this Ward I did not hear or see any patient actually benefiting from the somber 'movie theatre' setting of electric shock treatments. This E.S Therapy that I experienced as an observer never appeared to have any beneficial effect, it quite simply seemed like an experiment into the unknown mysteries of the brain. Psychiatrist would note in the patients chart, 'E.S.T. no change'. This treatment sometimes going on for months appeared to have no effect, but there may be somewhere out there that had success.

But what are the long-term risks I wondered?

Doctor John Ronald Andrews' Grand Rounds seemed like a bizarre tour into a prison-like maze, or the dungeons of a Medieval Castle, where tunnels led into other tunnels. The tunnels, or actually corridors, were badly lit, empty and quiet before he arrived. Rolling the keys around his hand and between his fingers, he chose the right key, opened the door allowing everyone in his entourage to *pass by him* before he would again lock the door satisfied that all was safe. He would then run to the front of the line pushing by them, even though corridor was packed, simply waiting for him. Now again at the front of the line our Captain of the Guard, with keys rolling around his hands marched to the next door. It was a pantomime in persistence. It was a ridiculous routine. It was not the 'Fast and Furious' pace of Medical Ward Grand Rounds, that other Consultants accomplished, but a slow, deliberate, repetitious and agonizingly period of two hours where Doctor Andrews essentially asked each patient the same question exactly as the last. How Psychiatry could possibly elevate itself from the annals of Renaissance times, I often wondered.

During my tenure in this glorious psychiatric hospital a remarkable event happened that apparently stunned and created considerable self-assessment for our Consultant, the leading Mental Health Advisor, Lecturer and Senior Psychiatrist Doctor Andrews, M.D., who in his earlier days as a Consultant had written a modern 'tutorial' book on the *'Benefits of Electric Shock Treatment or Electro-Convulsive Therapy, on Catatonic and Acutely Manic patients'*.

This Incident that would keep the whole hospital chatting about it long after it occurred seemed quite noteworthy, for all Student Nurses it was really amusing! Dru Tyrrell was my patient up in the Electro-Convulsive Therapy shock treatment Ward, where as usual, I inserted the tongue depressor and airway then watched the Resident Anesthesiologist inject the narcotizing drug and the patient slept. Doctor Andrews placed the electrodes one on each temple and delivered the electric shock to this tall, quiet fellow. The shock voltage increasing with each successive treatment, since from the last treatment there appeared to be no essential improvement in his condition. I remember his body go into a rage of physical convulsions, and Doctor Andrews remarking that this was his tenth shock and by now *should* be showing some modicum of improvement, apparently this young man did not seem to be progressing, I curiously wondered what a 'Modicum' of improvement might look like for Dru?

The patient's diagnosis on admission some six weeks previously was 'Catalepsy of Recent Origin'. Reviewing my own text book later and re-emphasized by Sister Winifreds explanation, was *a 'state of psychosis with puzzling physiological characteristics where there was no response by the patient to any external stimuli, including the muscular strength and rigidity of limbs that could be put in any position and remain statuesque there'.*

This Catalepsy condition is also known to occur in patients with Epilepsy as well as Schizophrenia, and to observe a patient in this cataleptic condition is quite saddening. Patients are locked in this state of their own prison. Nothing appears to penetrate their facade; their heads hanging down on their chests, their arms and hands held straight out in front of them with fingers widely spread, extending their reach. When sitting, their legs could be stretching straight out, not to the floor but appearing to be held in space by some mysterious force.

In fact, this was one of the cataleptic positions I had seen Dru display, and he had already been in that position for three hours! This was certifiable, 'a nut job' to some of his fellow patients! This fine physical specimen of a man, especially obvious when he removed all of his clothes and without them he was quite muscular. He looked to be in good physical health, and when Dru Tyrrell was dressed he wore his own tartan shirt.

Finally, after tearing several hospital gowns his family had brought him his own favourite Highland Green and Blue Tartan shirt of the Argyle and Sutherland Highland Regiment. Apparently he had loved the spirit of this proud Regiment and all their Scottish history as well as the long list of battles they had fought. Dru's Grandfather had been in the Argyle and Sutherland Highland Regiment in the First World War, and been recognized at Sterling Castle-the Regimental home-for his bravery. Below his proudly worn shirt he wore the usual striped hospital pajama pants, but he would carefully fold up his pants until they were just under his knees, like short pants. He may have been trying to recreate a kilt to go with his green tartan shirt. Since his admission no one had been able to break into his quiet world. In whatever position we would find him in, his muscles taunt and un-relaxing, we would feed him and he would swallow the food and seemingly drink whatever was offered him without any problems. He was actually easy to feed, it wasn't our words that encouraged him to eat or drink, and it was probably the taste of food on his lips. Inside his own strange, perhaps mysterious world where he was presently hiding he still seemed to have a strong sense of surviving, since he always ate everything on his plate- that observation was simply made. He certainly was very well nourished.

The night of Dru Tyrrell's glorious, rambunctious adventure, which was actually reported upon several days later in our local newspaper, happened on a perfect dark cloudy sky. No moon, just dark heavy rain-laden clouds. Dear Dru was not as lost in this odd world as we all had believed, for this was a well executed and planned escape, and it required a modicum of perfect timing. Like most of the other Wards in the hospital, the Ward's lights were out except for the one small lamp shaded light on the nurse's desk in the center of the Ward. That night, as all nights on the Psychiatric Wards, the one 'floating' Student Nurse would relieve each Ward's nurse for their meal break-but more frequently than not, the nurse doing the meal breaks would try and do two Wards at the same time. This unapproved, but possibly overlooked inappropriate behavior had been going on as long anyone could remember and nothing had ever happened that would cause alarm. But this night was going to be an exception! During this dark, cloudy moonless night, in the midnight hour, the Student Nurse sent to float and relieve Dru's Ward nurse got the brief report that everyone appeared to be sleeping. Indeed no one moved, the Ward was silent except for snores and regular breathing rhythms of the patients, all was as peace. Almost as a film screen script would sequence events, the relieving nurse left Dru's Ward to go and chat with a nurse on the opposite Ward across the corridor, this escapade now required that both Wards locked doors be left open therefore all the attention would be on the doors. Since no one was expected to die, have a seizure or crate a tantrum the nurse left the Ward at restful sleep.

On cue as the movie director would create Dru got up and out of bed silently and as always, dressed in his Scottish green tartan shirt and pajama pants, then put on his slippers. He had obviously observed that his neighbor's bed was directly underneath the window, which under usual circumstances required a six-foot stepladder just to climb up to the windowsill. Dru very ingeniously moved his own empty bed toward the center of the Ward, then pushed his neighbor's bed carefully and quietly into his bed's space, not disturbing this patients sleep. Dru's own empty bed he pushed under the window then he carefully turned the head of the bed to the floor with the foot of the bed now almost reaching the window. These were heavy cast iron frames and were meant to last for centuries! The bed, with the mattress tied to the frame, was now looking like an oddly shaped stepladder, his intention. The nurses chair from the center of the Ward, he pulled it over to become the first step, and from there Dru could climb up to reach up and over the narrow ledge of the sill, putting enough pressure on the windows locking latch, which broke from rust and years of never being used. Once the latch was separated he then used as much force as he could to open the bottom half of the window. This done he must have used the top of the mattress which may have broken away from its ties and doubled over the chair, this probably happened as he was struggling to break the window latch or push the window open using his legs for leverage against the mattress.

Now the mattress was nicely doubling over, which gave Dru the opportunity of step number two. Not a sturdy step but never the less another nine inches of leverage enough to open the window wide and climb on the narrow ledge. Whether Dru simply sprang from the ledge or lowered him-self down hanging on to the window ledge, then letting his body fall, we never quite knew. Outside, the fourteen-foot drop from the window to the ground had been broken by the Privet hedge, which surrounded the hallowed halls of this inner sanctum of the Fortress. The Privets were broken, but apparently Dru was not!

Perhaps Dru had carefully followed the script of the book, 'The Great Escape' the true world war two story, from 1944, of the escape against insurmountable obstacles from a well-guarded prisoner of war camp called Stalag Luft II, by British and Allied Airmen. Or perhaps he was a fan of the romanticism of that great historical novel *'The Count of Monte Cristo'* by Alexandre Dumas, and that fantastical escape. We had no indication where he had gone, he had left no belongings in his small beside cabinet and due to the blackness of the night it seemed, he had been swallowed up into those dark shadows of the town. He had truly disappeared from everyone's view!

No one saw him leave this hospital grounds, no one saw him on the streets by the hospital or in the town. Once it was discovered he was missing, and this was not done till four am in the morning when the Student Nurse did a cursory walk around the sleeping patients to find a bed frame up against the wall with its inhabitant gone! Nursing observation not a key process this night! The open window suggested that it was pointless to search the Ward, the corridors or its offices. Dru was gone, creating yet another masterful mystery. The Ward Sister, Mr. Larry Winifreds, and Matron and our *rolling key's* Leading Psychiatric Consultant Doctor Andrews were all called and all arrived. The police were called and they arrived with a couple of detectives. The only report that actually became the official record was that of the poor Student Nurses; the one who was there for the full shift and the Student Nurse who was relieving him for his lunch break. Both Student Nurses were charged with the responsibility of *'losing a patient'*. (It may have been kinder to state that these two Student Nurses were actually responsible for bringing back sanity to this patient!)

Within a week after Dru's successful *great escape*, the windows throughout this sober building were checked to make sure they could not be forced open, but those that could be opened, were repaired with new screw locking mechanism. Dru's photo, one we got from his family was published in our local paper for a full week, asking-but more like, 'pleading' for any information leading to his whereabouts. No one ever called. The general population were probably more amused by this remarkable escape, and more likely than not, wished him well. I know that all of the Student Nurses reveled in Dru's patient escape stunt. We tried to guess if he was still in the area hiding in some farmhouse, or perhaps he had been given a lift in some long distance lorry and was by now in those purple heather glens of the northern Sutherlands and seeking those Highlanders.

For us, Dru was a Hero. Dru did not want any more of those electric shock treatments he had had enough. No more interviews, no more being fed like a child, and no more questioning from Doctor John Ronald Andrews; and whether real or imagined, his Catatonic days seemed like they were over, and he was free of our Mental Hospital. He may remember his Psychiatric treatment and his brain being pounded by jolts of electricity, and his journey to freedom, a story for his children to come!

In my last year, Doctor Andrews still had lecture time for us, his topic of Psychiatric teaching ranged from the simple to the truly bizarre. Simple Psychiatric Diagnosis-he believed was never simple. Each category needed to be completely distinguished from the next. He had no doubt about his own competency to diagnose a true mental disease from a state of exhibitionism or intense situational behavior. These might be differentially diagnosed in the *'Diagnostic and Statistical Manual of Mental Disorders'*, or indeed the more widely recognized treatise, the *'International Classification of Disease'*. This 'ICD' was being recreated under the guidance from the World Health Organization, where from our good Psychiatrist's point of view, they were 'in need of his help and input to get it right'.

He truly believed his own unique competency was at a far higher level above these Psychiatric Internationalists'.

Encoding language, he taught us, was a primary characteristic of Mental Health, as an example, through the words used to 'encode a thought' as a 'phoneme' where the smallest unit of a language determines the clarity of meaning and these speech sounds, divide one word from another, simple as b's and p's, therefore simple communication understood. Similarly in this psychiatrists' mind, the linguistic element of a 'morpheme' where a word, 'mad' for instance, cannot be broken up into a smaller word that would have the same meaning. Mad it would remain!

Doctor John Ronald Andrews's lectures were always full of these fine explanations, seemingly great proof of his own academia, but puzzling for some of us. His parting lecture, I remember well, from a communication point of a view it seemed the wisest piece of common sense from all of his other lectures. He said, "Keep communication to its most simple principle, encode your thoughts, express them clearly into words, so the person hearing them can recognize both the symbol idea, hear the specific word sounds, identifying both and so it uncodes the full communication. This simple mental function clearly expressed the ideas of phones and morphemes. Remember them", he admonished us!

Doctor Andrews's lectures were generally enlightening; I enjoyed his 'no-nonsense get the information out style'. But then we had to try and to recompense his lecture ability and characteristics, against his bizarre and often odd behavior and certainly peculiar mannerisms of his actions on the Mental Wards as well as his dealing with patients and staff. Two different 'characters'; I wonder, does that require further investigation?

My Student Nurse colleagues and I decided that we should give him-whilst we were on the Mental Wards, a provisional diagnosis of 'situational schizophrenia,' and for the time being, we would delay the Electro-Convulsive Therapy, electric shock treatment, we had amusingly decidedly to treat him with. But for now, he was simply lost in his bifurcating worlds of fine lectures on one side, whilst on the other, a strangely mad or eccentric character, with unfathomable actions on the patients' Wards.

Whether he ever saw the drama of 'losing a patient', Dru Tyrrell, as a failure in his practice, or I wondered, did he secretly believe that the Electro Convulsive Therapy to Dru's resilient brain actually healed him? When anyone asked him if he believed Dru was healed, and he simply wanted to leave without an official discharge, Doctor Andrews would frown, then shrug his shoulders.

Dru, I hoped would be hunting deer in the early morning mists as the heather slowly showed its deep hue of purple on the side of some craggy Glen in the land of the north west Scottish coast of Sutherland and he deserved to wear a fine heavy woolen kilt.

CHAPTER 12

GERIATRICS

Victorian Melodies and Wheezing Old Geezers

Geriatrics, for me was lots of fun. Great and enduring Basic Nursing Principles. The care we delivered to these lovely old Geriatric folks was excellent, the best that could be delivered. If anyone chose not to like this wonderful Geriatric Hospital within the Fortress complex where it had, instead to be endured, it was probably a miserably tedious, monotonous and dull time. But it wasn't for me!

I learned a lot about roughly-yet tenderly, delivered compassion and an aspect of *'love'* that I had never thought or contemplated before, but it was there. It was the finest loving care, perhaps due to the nature of these Geriatric Wards and the wonderful people that worked upon them. I learned too, about being able to crack a smile on some old geezer who had decided he had come to this Geriatric place to die. Here, these Geriatrics patients did not come here to die, even though the bodies in which they lived, were frequently withdrawn into a mystical fog and more often than not, their limbs were tightly contracted into their bodies. Their prospects of being well cared for on the 'outside', especially if they were incontinent of both urine and faeces was very slim.

Aging carefully for many of these lovely old geezers before they got here, was not a consideration.

In spite of all the constant problems of aging and the ill health that generally comes with it, this Geriatric Hospital was alive with a whole Medical and Nursing Staff that thoroughly enjoyed this 'calling'. Making these patients feel alive again we brought smiles to their previously grim, tired faces, but most of all this Geriatric Hospital gave superb care to each one of these souls who had believed their life was over.

No patient in this hospital had a bedsore. Not one! They frequently came into the Hospital with various stages of bedsores, but under our care, they healed. No patient was ever allowed to even have the suggestion of redness on their bottom, heels, shoulders or elbows, absolutely no pressures sores!

This was the finest quality of basic nursing care I was ever to observe, and to be a participant in that arena care with its knowledge lasting a lifetime.

Our Gerontologist was quite odd, but the least odd of all the other Consultants, and he too was quite brilliant. He was a funny, kind and wise man, and occasionally he would express all of these traits at any one time, but generally was in one of these moods as he made his Grand Rounds. He was actually a local lad, being born in this town of ours to a missionary couple that had some years ago returned from living in the Philippines. They had returned from overseas because of his mother's pregnancy and because her father was the Professor of Gynecology at Birmingham University and Senior Consultant Gynecologist in the Birmingham Regional Hospital system. So it was appropriate that the Father of the Mother to be wanted to be the Physician of her care, as well as the Obstetrician who would delivered her child, his grandchild. Perhaps it was the heritage of this family back-ground that gave our Geriatric Consultant his behavioral characteristics of warmth and gentle caring, which he displayed during his consultations and patient rounds. He called this Geriatric Hospital his own. This was Mr. Edward Potter, Consultant, Doctor and Man-about-Town. In his younger school days, he was Captain of his school Football Team, as well as the school Cricket Team, he was a long distance runner, avid bicyclist and with all these attributes he was indeed an accomplished athlete, and he was proud of it, he had no interest in Football, he had said.

I loved this character of a man with his still noticeable local Lancastrian accent. Even though he was Under-Grad and Graduate of Cambridge University, he did residences in Internal Medicine and Psychiatry at London University Hospital and further residencies in Gerontology in Birmingham and Edinburgh.

In spite of the finer elocution, enunciation and the distinctive diction of Cambridge and London, Doctor Potter held on to his local accent and its intonations. He may have made a specific mental decision not to lose his accent, since most of his patients would come from the surrounding communities of the Fortress Hospital and his communications of speaking and hearing were in harmony with theirs. Of course, it was possible that a patient from some other part of Britain or overseas would eventually be his patient, but for now he was a Lancashire Lad.

To reach his office, which was to the right side of the main admitting and reception offices, and going down to his office, a short corridor and upon the walls were hung drawings and photographs of historic athletic significance and prowess. There was a photo of Edmund Hillary who reached the summit of Mount Everest with his Sherpa guide Tensing Norgay in 1953. There was a large framed photo of Jesse Owens, that famous Black American runner, winning at the 1936 Olympic Games in Berlin, Germany. An event that Hitler wanted erased from German memory. And I remember a photo on that wall next of the one of Jesse Owens, that had recently been placed there, that of Roger Bannister who in 1954 had become the first known person to run a mile in under four minutes. Both Hillary and Bannister had been knighted, so now they were 'Sir Edward and Sir Roger'. It seems that Jesse Owens, an American; missed out on knighthood, had he been born in Britain he would have become Sir Jesse.

In Doctor Edward Potter's office hung more drawings of athletic strength and energy, but the largest and by far, in the best gilt edged frame was a beautiful reproduction of that very well known painting of the *'Battle of Trafalgar'*, where the English Admiral, Lord Horatio Nelson and his British Seamen and ships soundly defeated the French and Spanish naval forces at Cape Trafalgar, off the coast of Spain in 1805. In that hour of victory Admiral Horatio Nelson died from a wound sustained during the battle, and as the painting depicted, Nelson died on the deck of his flagship 'Victory' of England but a loss to the British navy. Lord Nelson's, now famous words, which inspired his Seamen and Marines with his dying words, *"England expects that every man will do his duty"*. They did, they won.

On a prominent place in an open space on the huge heavily made, dark walnut brown book shelves, was a small silver coloured trophy in the shape of a Cup and below the Cup was a Shield that was emblazoned with the name 'Edward Potter' and a line under that which read 'County School Finalists', and below that, *'Winners'*. This was the only memento that he had brought to his office from home. The final Winners of the Cup were for the eleven year olds, which apparently was the beginning of his trophy collection in later life.

Behind the door of his office hung a dark gray-black suit, it was complete with a waist coat, a carefully folded handkerchief protruding artistically from the jacket's top pocket and around the jackets neck was shining silk tie of a light silvery blue colour. To everyone who worked in this Geriatric hospital no one had ever seen him wear this suit. Perhaps it too was a trophy. Nobody asked 'why' and Doctor Potter never told why. It was simply waiting for some yet unknown event, an occasion or some future celebration.

Doctor Potter's daily dress was the light brown corduroy sports jacket with leather elbows and a strip of leather showing at the collar, he wore light checkered shirts bought from Marks and Spencer's, he had told someone at an earlier time, that 'Marks and Sparks' always had the best shirts. On duty at the hospital he did not wear a suit. Daily, he wore only a shirt and a military striped Yellow and Red tie of the Lancashire Fusiliers, and his well-worn dark brown trousers. His choice of footwear was boots, brown boots with rubber soles, not an uncommon sight with some of our physicians. A peculiarity of his dress was the strip of material he had sewn into his shirt at the left breast pocket. The strip of cloth had a buttonhole firmly attached to a fine red button, which a seamstress had sewed. This strip of cloth was made into a loop, upon which he hung his stethoscope, "easy access" he would frequently remark, as he struggled to release the button, or the stethoscope.

Doctor Potter was of average height, had no extra weight on him. He moved with nimbleness as he led his entourage every morning to see every patient. There were two hundred and forty patient equally divided into male and female. He never missed a patient and spoke to every one of them, most answered him back but some did not. Those patients who did not answer verbally, he would go around the bed to get their eye contact, perhaps he was stubborn, but until they made some, any audible sound he would not leave that bedside. Only rarely did he leave after much coaching, concluding that the patient had a too powerful sleep medication, or had had a probable minor cerebral vascular 'accident' a CVA.

Every patient was asked the primary leading question every day, *"Had your bowels opened today"?* This curt short question was asked in a very clear precise way that every patient in the Ward could understand and hear it, knowing it was coming to them too! The question was repeated twenty four times at least the number of patients in each Ward so every patient knew what was coming, even if the patient was too slow to answer. Sister Gillian Holt, having the patients chart and checking the nurses notes would reply, "Yes, Doctor he has", or "No" and Doctor Potter would smile approvingly to the 'yes', or quizzically frown, if it was a 'No' then he would further question Sister Holt to find out how many days it had been without a BM, a bowel movement. It could mean an extra dose of Senakot, or Cascara, or an enema if the patients had no BM's for three days.

The Geriatric Hospital was divided into two separate half's; each half with their own separate staff. One side had the Consultant Gerontologist, with the House Resident Gerontologist on the other. Each side consisted of two floors, twenty-four male and twenty-four female beds, on the ground floor, and this was repeated on the second floor. There was also an Annex of 12 beds on each floor for 'overflow patients' if needed, essentially each side was a mirror image of the other. So it can be seen that Doctor Potter asked his 'bowel question' a lot of times before he got through all of his one hundred and twenty patients at full complement, perhaps he dreamed of bowels and intestines, enemas and soapy water!

During Doctor Potter's classroom lectures, he talked without fail about bowel movements. I distinctly remember, even today, that the overwhelming key to good health, mentally, physically, emotionally was to have a BM every day. He shared that the body's ability to maintain all of its electrolytes and bodily fluid balances were to guarantee that no part of our body was ever dehydrated.

Both problems with Diarrhea and Constipation are the key Electrolyte disturbances in all body functions. Of course, there are times when Diarrhea is a natural result of the body trying to rid itself of some gastro-intestinal bug or irritation, but creates huge amounts of watery stool flushing out the bugs. This is natural, so fluid intake becomes a vital necessity from this event.

Constipation by comparison, creates dehydration within the bowels. Fluids are removed from the bowel and stool becomes hardened and difficult to remove or evacuate. But, it must be removed by using medications of Senakot or Cascara; and if they don't work, then enemas or even manual removal is employed, and there by hangs a tale!

I know that tale. Manual removal of rock-hard impacted faeces is difficult for the nurse and painful for the patient. I did this distasteful duty a dozen or so times during my Student Nursing days on the Geriatric Wards. But this task was a very important part of keeping our patients healthy, and gave some of these elderly folk the opportunity of responding in the affirmative when Doctor Potter asked his key to life question of, 'bowels open'? Even today, I want to be able to answer in the affirmative for myself!

Sister Gillian Holt who was beloved of everyone was also a local girl. Having done her own Nurses training years ago at our Fortress Hospital for she too believed this Geriatric hospital within the Fortress complex was *hers*! *This* was her beloved Hospital! She was a buxom lass, but she could move anywhere with the ease of a Ballroom Dancer doing a Quick Step around beds, tables and a myriad obstacles. Our Sister Gillian Holt was in complete command of half of the Geriatric Hospital with a total of 120 male and female patients. She had grown upon 'the other side' of town from the

Fortress, so from the neighborhood in which she lived she could look down and across town, then up the hill on the far side of town, to where the dark outline of the Hospital Fortress stood mighty in its silhouette, a dark ominous character against a lighter coloured sky.

Sister Holt had a jolly, warm and loving personality. Everyone who came into contact with her would always remember, and remark how perfectly suited to this position of responsibility she was; as she handled times of sorrow, times of frustration, or hostility or even discipline with gentle care and understanding. If circumstances called for tact or patience as a family of a Patient whose aggression was coming to a boiling point, or some visiting Physician's misguided short temper Sister Holt would, with metered calm maturity bring them back to a peaceful understanding. She was a genius at conflict resolution and kindly persuasion. She had won many imaginary trophies year after year for *'the Ward Sister most likely to receive a Knighthood'*! Voted by her staff and the relatives of patients who wished to recognize her superior Nursing Skills.

Perhaps it was the unknown officials who recommended 'Knighthoods', but we knew they had yet to meet our Lady Sister Gillian Holt.

I remember my first meeting with her and an instantaneous smile crossed my face-for she wore her lovely Sisters Nursing laced Cap at a rather dramatically odd angle. It looked, no it was cock-eyed. It looked like she might have spent a night on the town with some rousting songs rocking back and forth so that the pins holding her cap in place had finally become loose and tipping her cap to one side.

However, in balance to her lop-sided, cock-eyed cap she always had both sleeves of her dark navy blue uniform rolled up to her elbows. This vision too, would suggest she had just completed washing the dishes after breakfast or lunch! This was no Lady; this was a genuine *Working Girl* not afraid of any work. Again, in getting to know this dear Sister of ours, I discovered quickly that she would help change beds of some incontinent patient's and whether it was a case of incontinence of urine or faeces, it never mattered. She could do everything she asked of others, and occasionally she would do the complete bed change and patient care on her own. This act alone endeared her to all of the Student Nurses and generated great respect from our geriatric Chief of Service Doctor Edward Potter. 'Sister Gill' as I, and everyone else called her, had an infectious laugh, and when she laughed her office or the Ward or the corridors echoed her joyful noise. Even though you may not have had any idea what the subject was, for you too would laugh in harmony. This place was fun. Sister Gillian Holt's lovely face was as round as her head. She wore her hair short and with 'bangs' falling over the forehead, she may have had very thin or fine hair that might account for her cap not being held straight on top of her head, but that mattered not! The cheeks of her face seemed to have an extra ounce or two of flesh and always appeared bright red, and when she laughed her checks wobbled, which in turn, somehow, made her bright blue eyes shine even more brightly. On one occasion, I had met her husband at the door of the Ward and he introduced himself as 'Betsey's husband' since I did not know any Betsey's, I had to further ask him who Betsey was. Expecting a surname he replied, *"Oh", I mean Betsey Holt, I call her Betsey because she once played a part in the play 'David Copperfield', and she was Betsey Trotwood, the temperamental and quite eccentric great aunt who in her kind hearted way comes to love, care for and eventually became David Copperfield's guardian".* She apparently loved that part of the Charles Dickens stories. After that long explanation, off I went to find our Betsey! Our real life nursing Sister Gillian who later explained to me-after I had asked her about her acting career, she replied that she thought she might even look like the 'Betsey' of Dickens story. Her husband had introduced an extension to the character of our leading Geriatric Ward, Sister Gillian, who we all already admired for her 'demanding-and getting-excellent quality Nursing Care'. Well, this lady probably had more hidden aspects of her character that we were yet to discover.

Her energy was endless, oft-times if we were short of staff, through an illness, she would continue to work long after she should have gone home.

Even working into the long evening hours without complaining. Her two Staff Nurses Natasha and Rene both ten years younger than Sister Holt were also a bundle of energy and good humour, the two of them giving so much extra of themselves, and extra hours. Sister Holt was the team to work for; I agreed whole-heartedly that these three, this terrific trio were Team One!

I met Matthew Blackshaw the very first day I worked on this wonderfully caring Geriatric Ward. He had been a patient there for the past six years, and he was completely bed bound. In all those years he had never been out of bed. He did not have a catheter to drain his bladder of urine, so even this single aspect of his care was a great attribute to his excellent care, No infection would come from a long term catheter in his bladder, which normally present a major problem of urinary infections. Matthew was eighty-three years old, his poor worn out body was contracted where his knees and legs were tightly folded up to his chest, the medically described 'fetal position'. He had no teeth-real or false, so his mouth appeared hollow as did his checks, this made his lips appear more sunken deeper into his mouth as though he was sucking lemons and this was accompanied by a low shrill sucking sound like nasty bat's in the belfry. This lovely old man was a bald as a bean, and besides his fetal position, his fingers were twisted and bent into tight balls of knuckles. Fortunately for all of us giving him frequent care, his small frame of just a hair below five feet coupled with his slight build he was very easy to lift him off the bed whilst we changed his bed linen. It was this careful attention of keeping all our patients dry and their pressure areas free from irritation or redness that almost guaranteed their continued general good health, with no skin breakdown, no tissue destruction, no MRSA! For Matthew on that first morning of mine, we met as I was doing the patient care rounds with one of the two orderlies; today it was Benjamin (Ben) Duxbury an elderly man of fifty eight who had worked on this Geriatric Ward of twenty odd years, so of course he knew all of these patients very well, and seemed to know all the gossip of the hospital in general, indeed this Ben character was a chatter box, and a great source of 'information'.

Amos's bed was the second bed in the Ward, so he was to be cared for, early in our rounds. Arriving at his bedside, the less than sweet fragrance permeated his surrounding; he obviously needed, as usual, a complete overall. Ben said smilingly, "This will be fun for you". Fun! I thought, how? Ben was a gentle soul and always had a smile for everyone and certainly for all our patients, but who was the actual beneficiary of this fun? Ben held my wrist, smiled even more broadly and said, "I'll show you, then you'll understand". The basin on the clean laundry bed-care cart or trolley was filled with warm water and the sponges we used for cleaning up BM messes, soap, plus the bottle of Methylated Spirits and the container of Talcum Powder and we were ready for whatever Matthew had waiting for us.

It was a warm summer morning so we did not need any extra covering for the patients when we stripped their beds and removed their pajamas, they needed to be stripped for us to give them a thorough cleaning and care, and to check all their pressure areas, besides which our mobile wheeled screens afforded privacy for each patient.

It quickly became apparent to me that there was a special bond between Ben and Matthew. Ben had warned me, before we began our rounds, "That both myself and my other Nursing Orderly partner 'might appear to be a little rough' on these old chaps, but in the end there is another unseen benefit for this nursing care". I wondered what purpose this explanation was for, and I soon discovered this *'little rough secret'*. If it had been the other orderly doing the rounds with me, Randy Telford it would have been the same explanation.

Now at Matthew's bedside, Ben's conversation was light hearted and kindly to Matthew, even though the topic seemed rather odd to me. Ben asked, "Hello Matthew, are you ready for your sweets' toffee"? Matthew replied by sucking more shrilly as he pursed his lips and since he was toothless, his lips became circular and seemed to disappear into his mouth, this must be his reply, perhaps for a 'yes'. Removing his covers, cleaning his malodorous stool off his buttocks and between his legs, then we made the bed up with laundry clean linen; so this simple task of cleaning, encouraging communication, and even patient exercise was the introduction of yet another aspect of my Nursing for Excellence in Quality 'Patient Care'.

To do this care for Matthew, and all the other patients, either equally immobile or with a better ability to move, the same dedication of cleaning and caring was done, even when some patients wanted to be left alone, or argued forcefully against getting care-they got care.

Matthew lying first on one side if his body then the other side, he looked pitiful. His back and spine had long ago been cemented into a messily curved shape, like a hunchback with his legs contracted up towards his poor pointed chin. His sadly fragile shape had lost all its muscles, it was just skin covering bone, thin lower limbs that were bent and held tight up to his chest. Is this a possibility of what could become of me in my old age, I wondered?

And I remembered a thought my Dad Eric, used to say when someone was criticizing someone less fortunate, it was *'There, for the Grace of God-go I'* It brings a personal consideration and reflexion to the moment!

As with all patients, like Matthew we now rolled him over to the unspoiled part of the sheet, with him supported by myself, Ben, after rolling Matthew could begin the thorough washing with soap and water on all his pressure points, buttocks, shoulder blades elbows and his heels. The soap and water was applied vigorously–helping the circulation and bringing some colour back into his skin. A clean sheet and a draw sheet were now applied to the side where the 'dirty' sheets were removed, and then the two sheets are pushed under the now clean Matthew so that I could now roll him back on fully clean linen. With the clean sheets now under Matthew we could now complete the 'pressure points' needing care. Matthew winched as he saw Ben reach for the spirits from the trolley. Is this the 'little rough care' about to begin, I wondered and frowned at Ben. Ben simply smiled at me and winked.

Odd I thought, but here comes the 'fun' that Ben was referring to in the process for good patient skin care having three separate stages, this is stage two, where the methylated spirits bring loud verbal exclamations from the patients after the soap and water cleaning. Matthew was now lying on his back with his lips drawn tight and that shrill sound escaping from his sunken cheeks it seemed to me that Matthew was perhaps mentally preparing for the next step or maybe he was dreading the anguish that comes with the next step! It came as a good dose of methylated spirits was generously sprinkled over Matthew's bony shoulder blades and his bottom, especially the protruding 'pointy' coccyx bone. Ben vigorously rubbed with the flat of his hand until there was no sign of the methylated spirits. Matthew gasped and whimpered and sounded like he was blowing bubbles, but his skin redden bringing back a healthy blood flow to nourish his pressure points, then Ben repeated the process to his heels and ankles and elbows. All this done, leaving Matthew breathing heavier respirations, leaving Ben to sprinkle talcum powder covering his back, shoulders and his heels-all the pressure points.

I gently rolled Matthew over to where he was now lying on his back and sitting him up supported by several pillows he looked almost content. Top sheets and counterpane folded at the uniform position on all beds, we were ready for the final performance of dear old Matthew. Surprisingly to me, Ben washed his hands then pulled a Barley sugar like toffee out of his pocket, tore off the toffee's wrapper and held this 'sweet treat' twelve inches above Matthew's face. This old man with his toothless sunken lips, hollow cheeks and bony face suddenly took on a brightened changed face whose sunken eyes now becoming wide open, remarkably alive and completely focused on that glorious sweet toffee inches away from his face. That succulent treat that would be his, he knew, but? His head and neck strained higher to get closer to this offered candy, although his arms, bent forever at the elbows with hands twisted and contracted into balls of bones with fingers buried into the palms of his hands he was making a heroic effort to stain all that he was capable of straining to reach that preferred reward, that early Christmas present, Matthew wanted that barley sugar toffee!

Ben and I watching these minute gyrations of whatever muscles he had left, and Ben smiled, but I secretly thought again, *'There, but for the Grace of God go I'*; I would do the same thing under these same circumstances, for I too loved all form of Toffee and Chocolate! The memory of my father flooding back again, wanting to make things right. So, Matthew straining upwards, Ben allowing the candy he held above his face to get even closer to his eyes and mouth. I was feeling a sliver of annoyance and of frustration, even a touch of anger with Ben tempting the impossible from Matthew. Then, Ben leaning now closer over the bed towards Matthew He whispered in Matthew's ear, "Ok you can have your Barley Sugar Toffee as soon as you sing your favourite song *'Come into the Garden Maud'*. This is my friend Harvey, and he wants to hear your song too, alright?"

This must have been a song from the shining times of long gone days in the early Victorian period, but here today and locked into the recesses of Matthew's mind and ears, this song I had never heard of, even the name Maud was an ancient name from the corridors of a stately castle or a character from a Dickens novel. Matthew began to mouth some words, but they were garbled, Ben gave him a sip of water to moisten his dry lips and mouth, and in a few moments Ben again encouraged him to try again. This time, the less than musical title line 'Come into the Garden' trailed off with a deep sigh. Another sip of water and the candy dangled even lower now just six inches from his nose, perhaps to the small morsel would be the greater encouragement Matthew needed. "Now Matthew as soon as you sing your favourite song for Harvey you can have your Barley Sugar Toffee, are you ready"? There was a whispered reply, and Matthew began with a surprising high-pitched strain of this old Victorian lyric, 'Come into the Garden Maud'. And he sang what must have been the first verse of this ancient song. I clapped in true joy; I smiled and said, 'Bravo', I was amazed. Matthew got his Barley Sugar Toffee and sucked on it with the relish of a hungry dog lapping and slavering over a bowl of newly offered favourite goodies.

This episode of perhaps unusual 'patient care', of getting static lungs to exercise, of muscles to strain and relax then strain again, and with patience, thoroughly monotonous skin care was to excel in the excellence of Basic Nursing Care.

To encourage a seemingly dormant non-communicating patient to come to life – exercise his flaccid muscles to have his neural functions both inside his brain and throughout his body spark back to life. Certainly this somewhat less than gentle, yet lovingly administered Nursing Care had brought Matthew back to life. Perhaps the Barley Sugar Toffee bought from the slim resources of Ben's own pocket was enough to give Matthew an extra lease on life. Over an eight-hour period Matthew would be changed twice and so got his Barley Toffee's. Other patients too, much like Matthew where they were unable to feed themselves, were sat high on their pillows so they didn't choke on their food and then they were spoon fed with a dedicated *compassion and patience*, by these Nursing Orderlies and Student Nurses.

This single attribute of spoon-feeding a patient who has trouble swallowing and an occasional patient with a neck and head that is constantly moving, is quite commendable, and I saw this often as the epitome of patience.

As a thoroughly qualified Nurse, this delivery of care in Geriatrics was part of the rigor of getting it right. I learned this gentle art, for I spoon-fed Matthew Blackshaw many times. Since he was tooth-less his foods were pureed, minced and mashed and amazingly he would always finish whatever was on his plate. I had fond happy memories of Matthew and his squeaky song of 'Come into the Garden Maud' for lots of years into my nursing career, he was one of many that I would sit by a bedside, and feed or read to, or per-haps deep into the night sit at the bedside listening to the tight and water filled lungs gasping for air as I talked about their family, or held their hand as we prayed together. With those patients with Pulmonary Oedema or Carcinoma of the Lungs I sat by their beds, as other Nurses would do, and if they had no relatives to sit with them, I would hold that cold, purple grey hand of theirs and chat about 'things' as they slipped closer towards their final breath. Yes, those times needed a special patience and I learned it from many people-both staff and patients.

Then there was Carla Fosterson. Carla had been on the Female side of Geriatrics for three and a half years and by all accounts she was one of the 'favourite' patient's of Sister Gillian Holt. Sister Holt was known to bring in from home her well read monthly magazine, *'Ladies Home Journal'* and not just this periodical, but from time to time she would surreptitiously place under Carla's pillow a Cadbury chocolate wrapped in tissue paper. All very clandestine but appar-ently a well know treat known by all the staff.

Carla, a jovial character whose lovely red chubby cheeks bal-looned round and expressive as she chuckled at some funny inci-dent or to a light hearted story. *She herself was to become her own light-hearted story*!

Her round face matched her cheeks, just as her rather short, plump body and stocky, fleshy arms and legs filled the bed. She was a few pounds overweight, but to watch her move up in bed then swing her legs over the side of the bed, you may have judged her a gymnast in her earlier years. But here she was ready for everything, especially at night and ready for bed, she would put on her lace nightcap, with red with white trim and for all intents and purposes she was Mrs. Santa Claus.

Before coming to our hospital she had been injured when she was trying to get off one of town's Double Decker buses. It was raining, and she simply missed her step and tumbled onto the pave-ment cutting her leg and tearing the skin above the ankle. It was the tibia, her shinbone that was badly bruised but not broken, she had bruised her knee and twisted her ankle as well, both of which were quite painful. The full amount of her weight falling onto her knee and ankle. Which was better than having a fractured hip no doubt. Apparently everyone at the bus stop had sprung into action upon seeing the blood from lower leg seeping over her ankle and shoe.

Remarkably, the bus she had tumbled off had pulled away, and another bus whose route actually stopped in front of the hospital quickly loaded her on and off they went without stopping. The bus drove past the front of the hospital going into the Ambulance entrance but not underneath the Casualty 'overhang' which would have taken the top part of the bus off! The bus company had called ahead to say the bus was coming, so the orderlies with their trolley were waiting for her and loaded her on to it immediately. Even in the driving rain Carla barely got wet in the transfer from bus to trolley, the orderlies and nurses getting her quickly into Casualty to be cared for and to get the bleeding stopped.

Carla had spent several weeks in hospital on the Surgical Ward, and after being discharged back home with her aging husband, had Home Visiting Nurse and Physiotherapist visiting her home weekly for three months. This indeed helped her get back much of her balance and standing as well as being able to make short steps. But her wound over the shinbone did not heal.

During Carla's recuperation time at home, her husband Andrew, her best friend helped her into to bed, and after making sure she was comfortable and didn't need anything, said his 'Good night and God Bless' to her, then he went to bed and never woke up in the morning.

Carla was heartbroken, her schoolboy sweetheart married her when he was nineteen years old and she was seventeen, now her beloved Andrew was gone and he had been a major crutch for her recent injuries, but more, he had been a great husband. He had been a cotton mill worker, a Foreman Weaver, in his time and he could fix everything in house and took care of the dog, they're back garden where his famous Roses and Rhubarb plants grew! Andrew had been a good Dad to their only daughter Natalie, and a doting Grandfather to their blond and blue eyed little girl, she was the pride and joy of both Grandparents.

Unable to cope after the loss of her husband, and not being able to reapply the daily dressings herself, or even cook for herself properly, and with her daughter Natalie working during the day, and Natalie's Flat itself was too small to accommodate Carla, she was admitted into Geriatrics and into the care of Sister Holt. Carla's joyful personality, with her almost immediate ability to settle into the Female Ward and all of its routine, had already become a 'favourite' *(although there were no favourite's)* of Sister Holt. Another reason Sister Holt liked Carla was the bright fun loving Granddaughter, Samantha who, when she visited Grandma she made every patient smile at her and they made her their friend too! Seven-year-old Samantha was the delight of the Ward every time she came with her mother Natalie to visit Carla. The little girl would go and visit all the patients who were wide awake, and ask them if they needed a drink of water or a drink of Lucozade from their bedside cabinet. This little girl was becoming a nurse herself as she would offer to go and bring a 'real' Nurse if a pain medication was needed, she would wander into the Sisters office and chat to whoever was there. The whole energy of the Ward was noticeably changed every time she visited. Carla was tremendously proud of her, and when she first arrived with Natalie, her mother she would jump up onto the bed and hug and kiss her rosy-cheeked Grandma, who in turn would coo and make noisy, slavery kissing sounds! At the point of my going over to the Female Ward to help a new patient on to the bed from the stretcher since she was grossly obese and the nurses needed extra lifting power, so I offered to go over and lift. In the next bed was Carla. She was everything I had heard about her. Carla even now suggesting a better way to lift this lady on to the bed, Carla, by now had become a body mechanics consultant. When the patient was tucked into bed and made comfortable I went to the side of Carla's bed and told her I had met her Daughter and Samantha who was singing a rhythm and skipping merrily away in the main hospital corridor as I was going off to dinner. A lovely discussion ensued with Carla, about the two stars in her life-Daughter and Granddaughter. When she had finished she asked me if I would do her a great favour, of course, I said, "yes". She explained that the 'bed cradle' the doctor had ordered and was on her bed was always falling to one side and slipping down the side of the mattress so she wanted me to pull the cradle out and press both sides a bit closer together so it would not slip. Since I couldn't get this solid, wide but smaller cradle to work properly I went to our supply room and found a higher but narrower cradle This was a perfectly rational, common sense thing to do, the cradle would rest more well balanced over her legs keeping the weight of the bed sheets off her legs, and it would also offer her a little more privacy from the beds in front of her across the Ward!

The job complete, and the new cradle back in place, with the bed sheets arranged over it, she was grateful, congenial and quite chatty, and I felt I had done a nice service for her. Little did I know that I was the pre-cursor, almost instigator to a clever plan that had already been hatched in Carla's very active mind! She may be bed ridden for now for too many months, but in a very unambiguous way she was laying a most careful delineated plan worthy of a Master Planner.

Perhaps she was a novelist, perhaps even a secret agent, but the best was yet to come. With the new technique of using ultra violet light on her wound, and keeping the weight of the bed sheets off, then spraying the wound when it was dry with a Sulphonamide powder, her wound had healed and new scar tissue was forming over it. The daily dressing had ceased earlier, three months ago, after our Gerontologist had wanted to see progress, and he was quite pleased, whilst doing his morning Grand Rounds. Carla had insisted on keeping her bed cradle 'for privacy', and since it seemed entirely appropriate the bed cradle stayed.

Even Sister Gillian Holt on her frequent daily visits to Carla had never suspected anything wrong or even sinister, everything appeared fine. Gillian still passed on to Carla those delicious Cadbury chocolate sweets and the Ladies Home Journal; everything was as it should be. Peace ruled in our world of Geriatrics.

The visits of Carla's daughter, Natalie with her curly haired blond daughter, our innocent 7-year-old Samantha continued with daily regularity from the time when Carla was originally admitted. It was probably this singular fact of seeing Carla's Daughter Natalie and with her always was Granddaughter Samantha. They were part of the daily routine, mostly coming in the evenings after Natalie had finished work, so they never seemed out of place. Everybody was kind and generous to both of them, offering Snacks, Soda or Sarsaparilla; the staff was always glad to see them at visiting hours, and in the afternoons on the week-ends.

Samantha was almost growing up in our Geriatric Ward; she was familiar with all the patients even bringing them flowers from the hospital gardens when they were in bloom. She did little errands for the patients, picking up or returning a library book or occasionally posting letters in the hospital mailbox. Both Natalie and Samantha knew all the Nursing Staff and the Resident Physicians, as well as the staff from the Kitchen and Dining rooms as well as the Security Guards on the Entrance Gates. In a well-mannered way Samantha used everyone's tile politely occasionally adding tit-bits about her Grandmother as, "My Grandma had a much better day than yesterday", or if we were carrying a tray or wheeling a trolley she would ask, "Is that for my Grandma Carla Fosterson?" I adored this bright little girl, for when I or anyone else spoke with her, she was well mannered, witty and quick with her answers. All this familiarity as we saw them visiting every day, gave us a sense of pride for this closely-knit family. The three of them really cared and shared a special loving bond between them, no other family members visited their relatives as they did, and it was a study in devotion and love.

An amazing discovery occurred one late cold January night. It was amazing because for three months not one person suspected or had any reason to believe there was anything out of the ordinary. A secret tightly kept.

But this unique event was most definitely out of the ordinary, it was bizarre by any accounts, and it stretched my imagination at the time and it still stretches my imagination. Had I not been there when it was discovered, I may never have believed it. Again, it was created and continued through this strong family bond of three Ladies of three Generations.

Whose original idea it was, whether Grandma Carla Fosterson, or Daughter Natalie or Granddaughter Samantha it verged on genius. Of course, the powers that were of Hospital Administration probably had 'administrative seizures' on the spot, and City, County and all Public Health division's, including the local newspaper-if everything had been revealed when it was immediately discovered-would have flooded into our Geriatric Ward. Pandemonium would rule!

The Female Ward had a Leader who carefully measured, and assessed, and contemplated carefully before proceeding, no acting on emotion here! We had the calm common sense and wise sensitive Sister Gillian Holt who, when finally appraised of this unique 'new' quality of her Ward, and upon arriving on the Ward she amazed everyone by her amusement and sensible decisions.

It was around eleven thirty that January evening when the Student Nurse who was sitting at small desk in the center of the Ward felt something brushing purposefully against her ankles and she screamed loudly! Almost all the patients were awakened by this instant loud, screeching scream, now fearful of some dark unknown menace. Awakened too, was Carla and she became very anxious, but at this point no one noticed her particular anxiety, she could hide somewhat behind her bed cradle. The Student Nurse ran to the main light switch and flooded the Ward with light. She slowly and surreptitiously crept back to the chair she had been sitting on at the small night table upon which the night-light shone. She looked under, over and around the table, then began looking between the beds close to the night table, nothing. She found the oversized flashlight in the desk drawer and searched under all the beds from her central position in the Ward.

She found nothing, and was now beginning to feel a little silly. After, fifteen minutes or so, now convinced that the 'rubbing' sensation on her ankles was perhaps her vivid imagination rather than reality, she encouraged all the patients to go back to sleep, as she again, turned off the main lights of the Ward. It was now just after midnight.

Peace prevailed again. But not for Carla. Carla had now come to the realization that her secret was now rapidly unraveling. The normally tight bed sheets at the bottom of the bed that helped keep her bed cradle stable and 'tent-like' on her bed, had become so loose that she could she see the Ward's night light through the interior of the cradle at the end of the bed. A calamity had begun that shook the hospital.

Carla's beloved Chihuahua dog that had been using the bed cradle for his secret kennel, and now the dog had gone!

Panic filled Carla's wakefulness, for now she was wide awake and began taking all the bed sheets off her bed and piling them on top of the bed cradle she moved her legs out of the cradle and over the side of the bed. Since her bed was close to the far corner of the Ward she hoped her movements would not alert the Nurse at her night table. Carla in her best quiet voice called the dog's name, "Lady, Lady, Lady" but no response, so her whispered calls to her tiny, short haired, smooth coated Chihuahua pet dog, grew louder, "Lady, Lady", she tried to whisper, but the calls grew louder!

The Student Nurse, now becoming very aware that there was a disturbance the far end of the Ward, in that darker corner area, someone was calling for someone! A problem she surmised; but for Carla now watching the nurse approaching her bed and thinking how she could still not be discovered, but Carla knew categorically both she and the nurse would be in trouble when the truth was 'out'. To help find her precious 'Lady' she knew she had to tell the whole story. When the Student Nurse learned she was also in charge of the 'pet shop' they both would have a dog problem!

And Lady was nowhere in sight!

Carla had no choice but to *'spill the beans'* and confess to her wildly illegal activity. Her beautiful friendly, quiet adorable pet Chihuahua dog had escaped, probably by falling to the floor through the end of the cradle and through the loose bed sheets at the end of the bed.

The Student Nurse stood at Carla's bedside, and was amazed that she had discovered a history-making event, but at the same time to be held accountable for not discovering the animal, a dog before now! No nursing books had ever described this event, nor had any lecture from the smartest of Consultants, and Nursing Tutor had never dreamed of this! Carla encouraged her not to be afraid because the dog had already lived here for just over three months. That loving pet Chihuahua had been either hidden in her bed cradle or cuddled in between pillows or her gown, from the time Carla's leg wound healed. Every person, Sister Holt, Sister Nicola Amber, Staff Nurses, Physicians or Consultants, Physiotherapists that had come to her bed, no one had the slightest indication there was more than one 'body' in her bed. There was never any doggie smells to suggest there may be a resident in the Cradle! So, Carla consoled the Student Nurse could not get into any trouble, since by inference, everyone should share in that guilt by association!

Now the secret had unraveled the immediate problem was where on earth had Lady gone? The nurse within a moment, realizing that the rubbing action she had felt on her ankles was the dog. She had certainly felt it, and noisily reacted to it but she had not seen it, so the hunt began. The Nurse did not want to turn on all the Wards lights again, so she used the flashlight. Wanting to keep her discovery 'secret' for now, besides which, she thought, it was not even one a.m. so there was no point getting anyone else involved till morning, and she still had no dog to prove anything. Lady was on the loose. Sensibly the Nurse asked Carla about the dog to get a better understanding of what she was looking for, but she was still anxious about the constant whispering by Carla and now herself, of 'Lady, Lady' over and over. She knew she was looking for Lady who had a smooth, pure white coat, with a black nose and pointed ears and large round black eyes, but she was tiny, only eight inches tall and barely weighting four pounds, her nature was quiet, friendly, and she rarely barked, although now lost she maybe whimpering. Carla told the Nurse that some people referred to this dog breed as a 'toy' dog. After sweeping the flash light under all the beds close to Carla's bed and finding nothing, Carla pulled a deep saucer from her night stand and asked the nurse to fill it with some milk also from her night stand and put in on the floor near Carla's bed and where she could see it, a temptation for lady. It was not until the Nurse reached the far end of the Ward from Carla's bed, at the entrance to the Ward where the sink was, with a towel rack and a rubbish container, and there was the whimpering elongated body of the white-coated Chihuahua. Hiding with her legs folded under her, behind the rubbish container. The nurse switched off her flash-light, and slowly bent down on her knees and quietly coaxing the dog, 'Lady, Lady, Lady' as she picked up the shivering, frightened white bundle of this tiny dog. After taking Lady back to Carla who was now completely relieved the dog was back in her care, had the bed made up again as before, with the bed cradle becoming the 'kennel'. Carla was now-rightly or wrongly convinced that all had to end well. Carla's family had no phone and it seemed foolish in the middle of the night to call out the police force to go and get the family, so that idea was on hold for now.

The Nurse had a major responsibility to tell someone and to help get the blame, if there was any, off her shoulders. With perfect luck, Sister Holt's colleague from the second floor of the Geriatric Hospital, Sister Nicola Ambers was the Hospital's Administrative Sister for the night. And she, like Sister Holt was a gentle mannered kind and understanding lady, who was also easy to talk to, and was not known to shout, so far so good. The Student Nurse called Sister Ambers office, and when she answered, spoke quietly with some trepidation explaining that a dog was in bed with a patient and after getting, "Oh my goodness, how, why, who", on the other end of the phone, the student went on to say that the patients foot cradle had become a dog kennel for over month! So our Student

Nurse was more relieved when Sister Ambers said she would come over to the Ward shortly.

Carla was already making plans by the time the Student Nurse came back to her bedside. The Student, now seeing the white coated Chihuahua against Carla's white night gown as well as the white pillows cases and sheets, realized how well the camouflage worked; it now became clearer how well this tiny dog could blend in with bed and occupant!

Carla had began bargaining with the Student Nurse to keep Lady till her daughter and granddaughter arrived at the evening visiting times, but the Nurse told her the dog would probably have to be gone from the Ward before the day shift arrived, and the two of them chatted until Sister Ambers arrived.

Calmly, Sister Ambers approached the bed at the end of the Ward where the bed cradle-kennel was outlined by her flashlight. The Student moved from the chair to let Sister Ambers sit down, and once sat down the patient and the Sister remade their acquaintances Carla now pleading for sympathy for Lady, the dog. Apologizing for 'not obeying the rules' by cleverly stating, 'how much help the dog had been in my rapid recovery'.

Sister Ambers had already made up her mind how to solve this curious but well executed deception of successfully hiding Lady in the bed cradle for the last three months, *under the nose of everyone!* But obviously, it had to end, and end within a few moments. Remarkably, it seemed only two or so patients were vaguely aware of the disturbance, but no one knew the actual cause of the commotion, so there were no further explanations needed for the patients.

Carla now in tears, clinging to her pet, kissing Lady on the head and nose knowing she had to let go; but not just yet. Sister Ambers plan was to let Carla keep Lady until around five thirty a.m., before the Wards early morning activity began. She would come back with a loosely woven basket with a lid attached with leather straps, from the recreation room, put some towels in the bottom of the basket and when it was time – pop the dog into the large basket and close the basket lid. There was plenty of airflow through the open weave so the dog could breathe easily and see outside. Just before six o'clock she brought the basket to be filled with Lady the, 'soon to be famous' white Chihuahua, to Carla's bedside where she said her tearful goodbyes to Lady, and popped her in the basket. Sister Ambers took her to the Administrative Office and awaited the powers to be to share the hospitals' star attraction.

Carla Fosterson at peace with Sister Ambers plan for Lady, but was sad that she had been caught, rather than found guilty of a major public health offense. Sister Ambers was actually very kindly going to drive the dog to Carla's daughter Natalie's home at the end of her night shift.

As the entourage of the Administrative Nursing and General Hospital Administrative staff arrived they were for the most part amused and amazed. Only the Matron, our highest nursing authority, didn't actually show one bit of amusement nor was she impressed by patient Carla Fosterson's stealth and 'cover up'. Her questions and *'grave concern'* was for the local or County Health authorities to hear of this escapade in *her* Hospital! We never knew whether this incident was ever reported to Public Health or any other authorities but once Lady had been returned home, eventually the story, the gossip of this amazing feat would be forgotten-by some.

Dutifully when Sister Nicola Ambers ended her shift she popped the open weave basket containing Lady, our Geriatric mystery patient into her car and drove to the home of Carla's daughter Natalie and granddaughter Samantha. All this time on the Ward the dog had never barked, whimpered a little bit, but did not bark.

Nicola Ambers knocked on the front door of Natalie's home; Samantha, who was just getting ready for school, opened it.

The child and the Ward Sister both recognized each other, but before Sister Ambers could say anything Samantha cried out with tears rolling rapidly down her face and calling, "Mummy, Mummy come quick it's about Grandma". Natalie rushed in from the kitchen, surprised to see Sister Ambers standing at the front door and before the Sister could say anything barely audible barking noises were coming from inside the basket, which she was holding. It seemed that same instant both Natalie and Samantha knew who and what was in the basket!

At this rare moment in all three of the lives dealing with Lady it was joyful, happy and yet sad that Grandma couldn't have her beloved dog Lady with her, never the less it was a warm reunion.

Sister Ambers learned that when Natalie and Samantha visited Bertha, it was Samantha that put Lady into a small cloth shopping bag, then took Lady out to the grassy areas where she would have her daily poop, pee and friskily run around getting her exercise. Lady was fed a few tasty morsels that Samantha had brought from home; and after a good running around, she would gently put the dog back into the cloth carrier bag and bring her into Ward again completely unnoticed.

This lovely family of ladies, Carla, Natalie, Samantha and Lady their cuddly female Chihuahua may well have served as a great fore-runner for institutions of the future caring for the elderly infirm. Especially for those facilities dealing with the memory care issues of Alzheimer's, Senility and Dementia. It was these long term care Institutions that would initiate the presence of loving, gentle dogs and cats to be a comfort and companions to those amongst us who are losing their memories of all they hold dear, for those patients have moved into complete helplessness into a world where there is no one, only silence.

So we need, no, *must have* a Nursing Staff that really cares, that can show warmth, compassion, patience and love, for Love Never Fails, guaranteeing that the Profession of Nursing will continue to be a bright light shining onwards.

And, *'THERE BY THE GRACE OF GOD GO I'!*

About the Author

John Harvey Greenhalgh, a Lancashire Lad, began Nursing as a 'Cadet Nurse' in 1954 at the age of 17. One began as a Student Nurse at age18. That year as a Cadet Nurse, learning the skill of sharpening needles and making sure the 'red rubber IV tubing' was thoroughly flushed out, as well as scrubbing bed-pans, bottles and kidney dishes then sterilizing everything, besides working hard at the basic Ward hygiene and housekeeping tasks. In the next three years as a Student Nurse, at a large Hospital complex in Lancashire, England, had the most incredible experiences of meeting and working alongside many wildly eccentric, bizarre, odd-or perhaps bordering on madness, Physicians and Consultants, yet were all quite brilliant! During this total 4 year period, Harvey learned what 'NURSING CARE' really meant. It IS the professional understanding of every aspect of high quality, unbeatable CARING, learned from those powerful Ladies in Navy Blue-the Ward Sisters; and of course the Patients he cared for with tenderness, gentle patience, increasing skill and even love.

After gaining his S.R.N., Her Majesty beckoned, so off into the Royal Air Force to do his 'duty' as a Nurse, that lasted 5 wonderful years, at hospitals in RAF Cosford, England; then to APL Hospital, Khormaksar, Aden, (now Yemen), Arabia; and back to RAF Hospital Ely, Cambridgeshire. Whilst in the RAF had the opportunity to do Nursing at a Hospital in Kenya. After returning to England, and wondering what happened to the Blue Skies and Sunshine of those far away places, emigrated to California, USA, and became a proud Yank. Obtained his R.N., B.A., M.A., and PhD. Going from

Staff Nurse, Head Nurse, Administrative Nursing Supervisor, and Assistant Director of Nurses. A life full of NURSING, with Great Care, and lecturing in California and the Philippines.

He would do it all over again! December 2014

Basic and Brilliant NURSING CARE.

This is a true glorious look at Medical Care, Par Excellence' Nursing Care & Caring. A compendium of incredibly eccentric Physicians and Consultants who cared for our patients during the 1950's in England in a hospital we referred to as, 'The Fortress'.

In the days where hospitals were sometimes called the 'Infirmary', Emergency Rooms were called 'Casualty', and where the Matron in dark green and the Sisters in deep navy blue ruled supremely. These stern disciplinarians of the hospital systems throughout Great Britain demanded and got the finest, caring Nursing Care for their patients.

This was a time when many of the Physicians came from generally wealthy families. They were not looking to 'make a fortune in medicine', but rather, theirs was more a desire to 'save mankind'. Perhaps it was this noble attribute that engendered their fascinatingly bizarre eccentricities. None dare call them Mad!

In those days, there was no 'use it once' then throw it away. Everything had to be washed, scrubbed, irrigated, sharpened and sterilized then used over and over. Especially the red rubber IV tubing and all those needles had to be sharpened by hand.

There were times of great joy, wonderfully happy and very humorous events as well as those profoundly sad and heart-wrenching moments. From Cadet Nurse to Student Nurse and so eventually up the ranks, what a great wondrous adventure it was!

I would not hesitate to do it all over again. JHG. S.R.N., R.N. etc.

FINEST NURSING CARE. ALMOST MAD, ECCENTRIC & BIZARRE PHYSICIANS. BEYOND SHERLOCK HOLMES EPIDEMIOLOGIST. SUPER SENSITIVE PEDIATRICIAN. MENTALLY CHALLENGED PSYCHIATRIST. BLACK CURLY HAIRED DIAGNOSTICIAN. FABULOUSLY 'OUT TO TEA' SURGEON. GASTRONOMIC-END EVENT-GERONTOLOGIST. BIZARRE, AMOST INEXPLICABLE DEATHS. UNIMAGINABLY BEAUTIFUL BABY & SPINA BIFIDA. SPINAL NEEDLE PLUNGING STUDENT NURSES. GREGORIAN CHANTING STUDENTS.

This book is written for

ALL THOSE WHO CARE for ANOTHER,

For those with Compassion, and a desire to give something more that a monetary reward may not achieve. CARING comes from so many avenues of life, and from many people. Family, Nurses, Doctors, Firemen, Policemen, Neighbors, Therapists of all descriptions, Those Teaching others how to 'do it right' for those who cannot, especially in Long Term Care and Geriatric facilities, or Alzheimer's-Memory Care units. And to Nursing Educators in University or Junior College, remembering how the very basics of care bring their own health and wellness, upon which is built a good healthy living and a long life.

To all those LVN's and Nurses Aides; so many of them over the years, that say when explaining what they do, "I'm just an LVN", or "I'm just a Nurses Aide".

Please, DON'T EVER SAY IT AGAIN! You are the eyes and ears for the Nurse and the Doctor, the Patient needs you, the Family needs you. Be the Best you can be!

CPSIA information can be obtained at www.ICGtesting.com
Printed in the USA
LVOW04s0606150115

422830LV00003B/3/P